Women of Silence

Grace Gawler

Women of Silence

The Emotional Healing of Breast Cancer

for all women interested in:

- Healing
- Prevention
- Understanding

  and
- Living Well

Live your truth and be yourself

Grace Gawler

HILL OF CONTENT PUBLISHING
Melbourne, Victoria, Australia

First published in Australia 1994
by Hill of Content Publishing
86 Bourke Street, Melbourne, Australia 3000

Cover illustration: "Night and her Train of Stars"
Edward R. Hughes by kind permission of Birmingham
Museums and Art Gallery, Birmingham, England.
Typeset in Australia by Schuurman Computer Service
Printed in Australia by Australian Print Group,
Maryborough, Victoria

National Library of Australia
cataloguing -in-Publication data

Gawler, Grace, 1953–
Women of silence
Bibliography.
ISBN 0-85572-254-1

1. Breast — Cancer.
2. Breast — Cancer – Psychological aspects.
I. Title
362.19699449

WOMEN OF SILENCE

Women of Silence, gentle and strong,
Tell me your path, where you first went wrong
Tell me your story, how you've coped with your life.
Tell me about all the trouble and strife.

I see how you've coped, withholding the pain.
I feel your soul weeping and yet you refrain
From sharing your losses, your grief's and your fears
But you know they multiply over the years.

Until one day your inner wisdom says "no more."
And you awake with a cancer, a fiery core
That's fed by a lifestyle out of control
Too much held too often, has taken its toll.

It's time to rethink, reassess how it's been
And develop a strategy previously unseen.
There is a way to heal with heart and great passion.
Let go of withholding—that was always your fashion.

Nurture yourself and make yourself whole.
Live your life fully and realise your goal.
Women of silence, gentle and strong,
Find the courage to heal, to sing your heart's song.

DEDICATION

"There is not one big cosmic meaning for all, there is only the meaning we give to our life ...

To give as much meaning to one's life as possible is right to me."

And so it is to me.

I dedicate this book in the true spirit of healing to my sisters with whom I share the path and journey of womanhood. Also to the many Women of Silence who have transformed their lives with dignity and wisdom and who have ultimately found their healing ... and the meaning of their lives.

Grace Gawler

Contents

PART THREE:
Appendices

Acknowledgements

The writing of this book has been somewhat of a surprise for me. For at first *Women of Silence* asked to be written, and in fact it came into my consciousness twice before I finally took up the challenge and put pen to paper. But it was not until a car accident gave me the "gift" of an enforced holiday and provided me with both the inspiration and the time, that the manuscript began to take form. It was as if all my years of experience were crying out to be birthed—all at once!

So, for me this has been an extraordinary learning time. To write a book which had no previous conception or planning in my mind seemed rather a daunting task, however, it began to appear inspirationally—often at times with a creative urgency. Sometimes it would come in pages or paragraphs, wherever I happened to be or whatever I happened to be doing! I just had to stop and write. Eventually, I arrived at a point where I kept writing, which of course disturbed my usual lifestyle and my work, but the sheer importance and urgency of this topic embraced my entire being. It was almost as if the angel on the cover was weaving some sort of wonderful magic, impelling me to birth this book as quickly as possible! The beauty and symbology of "Night and Her Train of Stars" seems to represent the positive side of nurturing and therefore the positive side of the breast cancer story. I feel her presence to be that of a healing angel for all those women who suffer in silence.

Obviously, writing a book in the above manner has created a few logistical problems and I have many people to thank for their help, care and support.

To Digital Australia, in particular, Cris Nicoli and Mrs. Misty Bunker, who provided me with my "intelligent friend," a Digital laptop, which readily converted my thoughts into text. Also Digital has generously provided much-needed equipment to The Gawler Foundation.

To Robert Kirby and John Huddle, who, as President and Treasurer of The Gawler Foundation, have wholeheartedly supported The Foundation's work, providing skill, expertise and a heartfelt commitment to the needs of cancer patients in the community—thank you for being there.

I have great appreciation for all the staff members at The Gawler Foundation who have taken on many extra responsibilities and workloads in my absence. A special thanks to Scott Crisp, Pat Beale, Kay Kelly, Lynette Archer, Maureen Van Der Linden, Lisa Burke and Howard Errey. Also to our therapeutic staff members, Bob Sharples, Trevor Steele and my husband Ian—a very big thank you for your energy in keeping the programs going and working extra time to allow me space to write.

And special thanks to my new friend and fellow therapist, Tara McKinty, whose timely arrival on Australian shores has been a great support to me.

I am fortunate to have the world's best as my publisher. Michelle Anderson at Hill of Content Publishing has supplied me with loads of enthusiasm, encouragement, support and trust in this project for which I sincerely thank her.

Olivia Bell from Australian Print Group—thank you for your patience and the wonderful printing, especially the superb reproduction of the painting of "Night and Her Train of Stars" on the cover.

Thanks also to the Birmingham Museum and Art Gallery and Birmingham City Council for their permission to use this most inspiring painting for the front cover and tape jackets.

Special mention and thank you to Graeme Burke from Village Roadshow, Showads Omega and Chanel Press who generously donated the design and printing for my tape covers and Breast Cancer Residential brochures.

Once you have put your heart and soul into producing a book such as *Women of Silence*, there come two crucial stages where you trust the content to be sculptured and formed into the finished book—a process which has been like observing a butterfly emerge from a cocoon. Firstly, my typesetter, Robbie Schuurman, whose high standard of work, combined with a friendly and flexible manner, has been truly a Godsend. Secondly, the editing process, which I regarded as a formidable task, saw my manuscript treated with the delicate care that was required so as not to alter the feeling and intimate nature of the text. I am pleased to say that my husband, Ian, filled this role in a caring, capable and loving way, in the midst of a busy work schedule, for which I am most grateful.

To Richard Osborne, RMIT Department of Medical Laboratory Science, a special thank you for his rapid replies to requests for literature referenced in the Appendix—Part III.

Also thanks to the Medical Journal of Australia for their permission to reprint studies also featured in the Appendix.

The Institute for The Advancement of Health provided me with enormous quantities of studies in Behavioural Immunity from their extensive publications, summarised by Steven. E. Locke and Mady Hornig-Rohan. Thanks, not only for their use but also in bringing this important work to the awareness of the medical profession. To Allan B. Chinen M.D., author of *Once Upon a Midlife*, who kindly gave permission to reproduce a story from his book—thank you.

With respect and thanks to the late Dr. Ainslie Meares and his personal assistant, Vere Langley, pioneers in the field of mind–body medicine.

To Norma, whose love radiates out to me wherever I am in the world and who always appears exactly when she is needed. Her wisdom, clarity and presence have provided me with strength and the attitude of the feminine warrior in completing this manuscript!

And to my dear friend, Dorothy Hall, who opened up the door to healing for me in another way—a woman of high integrity, good humour and a wisdom that has encouraged me to practise the *Art of Herbal Medicine* in the traditional manner.

To Pat Coleby, salt of the earth, tower of strength. Thanks for being there.

A big thank you to my four children—Rosemary, David, Peter and Alice—who have understood the importance of this project and have been prepared to be more self-sufficient so that I could take the space to make it happen.

Special thanks to Peter and David who helped me with computer printing and other keyboard work.

The stories appearing in *Women of Silence* are factual, however, patients' names have been changed to respect their privacy. Thank you all for the trust in sharing your life journey with me and with other women, who at this time are so in need of hearing about the positive side of breast cancer. thank you to every woman who has shown the way for others to follow, because that's what it is all about.

Introduction

You may be surprised by the insights and concepts that are broached on the following pages. Associating women's emotions with the onset and progression of breast cancer may be a challenge for some women. For others it may come more as a relief; linking as it does feelings that they have felt inside but found no avenue to express.

Having started an innovative cancer support service with my husband Ian in 1981, I can draw on many hundreds of case histories of women with breast cancer. As a result I feel I have something important to say to the women of the world about how they might live, connect with their inner potentials and in so doing build on and improve their own lives and the lives of their daughters.

As a woman I have been touched deeply by the lives and stories of so many women affected by breast cancer. As a wholistic healer, it would not be appropriate for me to maintain silence or withhold the knowledge I have gained. At this moment of writing I am thinking about all the women who have journeyed in and out of my life over the past 20 years; each one of them being like strong threads in the finely woven fabric of life. Some have survived with immense dignity and courage. Others have died with immense dignity and courage. It is in honour of these women's journeys that the book is written.

These women's support for me in writing this book actually enabled me to "put on my warrior shoes" and get on with it. Anyone who has written a book will appreciate what I mean! With my family of four children aged from 10 years to 16 years, Foundation commitments and farm duties, it has not been easy! However, like the process of healing, it has required enormous amounts of self discipline, perseverance, determination and energy as well as learning new skills such as making friends with computer technology. Producing the book has been like the birth of a child—it has involved a creative process, hard work and finally the expulsion into a physical form of something that has been tenderly incubated inside for some time. It was a fascinating insight when I realised that in order to complete the final draft in peace and quiet I had indeed moved my entire writing operation into a building on our farm affectionately known as "the shed." This is the place where I had given birth to three of my children. How symbolic that I should be birthing my book in that same space!

The book is divided into three parts:

PART ONE of this book will deal in depth with the emotional aspects of a woman's life in relation to disease and healing.

This is an area often neglected in conventional medicine as we know it today. In my own clinical work with cancer patients, especially women with breast cancer, the similarities in their emotional life histories have been too obvious to ignore. This is the hidden side of cancer. Although there are visible lumps on and in the body, these symptoms may actually have their origins within the soul, where the creative threads of life dwell. When there are blocks in the creative flow of a woman's life and when the expression of that creativity is blocked, her creative threads can become knotted, knotted into what are unhealthy "knots of the soul." These "knots" are formed by frustrated emotional energy at a very deep level of the psyche.

Interestingly, women dealing with breast cancer, almost always have a history of unresolved emotional pain throughout their life. Commonly also, about eighteen months to two years prior to diagnosis a key traumatic event took place in their lives. Many women have told me that about this time they either underwent a major change in life circumstances which they had great difficulty coping with, or they suffered a major trauma of some kind that "knocked them off centre," shocking them to their very marrow.

When you drop a stone into a pool of water there is a ripple effect—circles radiate out across the water. Using that analogy I believe that many of the modern orthodox and alternative treatments for cancer are focused on the "ripples" only. To me it appears that they are failing to see that the ripples are a consequence, or a symptom, of a greater block and that block is like the original stone that was dropped into the water. If we observe this mechanism and can find the central issue that created the pattern, we can understand that the ripples of our life are not causes but consequences. By going back to the stone, the originator, we help to fully heal the ripples. This then becomes healing from the inside out.

Patients who consciously participate in their own healing with this type of idea as their premise, tend to experience a marked increase in the effectiveness of other healing modalities. This applies whether it be chemotherapy, radiotherapy, alternative remedies or a combination of them all. When the patient sees for themselves that there is some rhyme or reason associated with their illness, a sense of personal empowerment is achieved. When this happens the patient becomes an effective participant in the treatment and outcome of their condition. This highlights the difference between being a victim of cancer or becoming a victor.

In other words women who take this view, move from experiencing their cancer as just plain bad luck to seeing a connection between the mind and the body and feeling empowered to heal. This new understanding emphasizes the importance of the role of the patient as a key player in their own healing. Doctors, Oncologists and Natural Therapists cannot switch on the "will to live" button. It is up to the patient to take that role. The will to live is born out of a strong desire that you do not want to die and is a survival instinct that is often motivated by fear. In the process of healing it is followed closely by the will to heal which is a condition in which fear is allayed, techniques for healing sought after and then an openness and readiness for transformational change becomes apparent. It is as if there is a bridge between the will to live and the will to heal. When you begin to cross it you can begin to transform your life through the illness rather than passively lose your life to it.

PART TWO of the book will deal with the practical details of breast cancer management. We will be considering this from the point of view of nutritional help, meditation instruction, stress management, dealing with any side effects of treatments, natural therapies and many facets of care. Issues relevant to hormones, osteoporosis, and coping with surgically and chemically induced menopause will also be discussed.

The information that I share with you clearly is not intended to replace any medical care and treatment that you may be having. Rather I hope it will give you understanding and clarity regarding your individual situation so that you are better able to develop a healing program that incorporates the best that orthodox medicine has to offer with the best of other complementary approaches. My hope is that the result gives you the best chance of survival and a better life ahead.

PART THREE of the book is combined as the Appendix. This section contains a cross section of medical and scientific literature which both you and your health practitioner can benefit from. Some are taken from orthodox Medical Journals—the type that your doctor would read. Others are taken from journals of Behavioural and Social Sciences, Journals of Mind–Body Medicine and other reputable Journals from around the world. Important too is the inclusion of The Gawler Foundation's submission to The House of Representatives Standing Committee on Community Affairs Inquiry into the Management and Treatment of Breast Cancer. This paper gives a clear understanding of the importance of Cancer Support Groups in Australia today and was composed by my husband, Ian Gawler.

Part One

"Women of Silence, Gentle and Strong..."

Chapter One

The Journey of a Lifetime

For over 20 years now cancer has occupied a major part of my life. During that time I have had contact with literally thousands of people affected by cancer. It has been a privilege to play a part in helping them to find healing and meaning in their lives. I have made many lifelong friends and also have the legacy of the life stories of those for whom physical healing was not attainable, but who nevertheless left this life healed with all unfinished business attended to. These people and their courageous families have been great teachers to me.

I have had a long term interest in the healing arts; but it was not until 1974 that my world suddenly took a dramatic change in direction. It was at that time that my good friend, work colleague and future husband, Ian Gawler, developed a bone cancer known as osteogenic sarcoma. As a result he had a full leg amputation in January 1975. I lived with and cared for him throughout that year and life began to resume some sort of normality. Our life together was to change more radically still, however, when in late 1975 secondary cancer was diagnosed. We were faced with a grim prognosis. Three to six months life expectancy. At this time, with no medical treatment available to offer curative hope, we set out as pioneers on a healing journey with fire in our souls and passion in our hearts.

Firstly we followed a dietary approach which seemed to us to make a lot of sense. Indeed a major part of our veterinary practice was involved with performance animals: racehorses, trotters and greyhounds who all required specialist nutritional help along with vitamins, minerals and trace elements. Their nutritional status was probably much higher than that of their owners! It seemed natural to us therefore that diet could help in the healing process.

At the same time Ian began to make the connection between his cancer and his own life as a high performance person. He regularly worked 80 hours per week, trained and competed in Decathlon, was involved in the local football team and was leading an active social life with "yours truly." Life was fast and fun; but insidiously stressful.

So the second mainstay of our approach to dealing with Ian's cancer became meditation. Ian attended regular sessions with Dr. Ainslie Meares, a Melbourne psychiatrist who had an intense interest in hypnosis and a type of meditation he called mental ataraxis. This was a technique of totally letting go—without the use of one's willpower, striving or trying. It led to a deep inner stillness. The return to the very centre of one's being. Ian enjoyed these meditation sessions immensely and would often spend up to five hours per day meditating. It gave him a focus and built our hopes.

Along with Ainslie's support, this intensive meditation sustained us through difficult times and seemed to be the only source of self help and positivity available to us.

Although what happened in Ainslie's rooms could not be termed a support group, Ian did make valuable connections with other patients attending at that time. Often members of the group would meet after meditation and their bonds were strong.

I began meditation too in order to support Ian. Although I had been skeptical at first; the theory made sense to me and I soon felt the benefit. I found Ainslie's assistant, Vere Langley, incredibly supportive. It was strange really as we had little verbal exchange but she added a strong and gentle feminine presence which somehow I felt able to draw upon. There were several women of substance who supported me along the way and she was one of them. Pat Coleby was another whose support kept my strength and courage alive through dark times. Pat knew at heart what we were up against as she had been through the cancer experience with her son. I remain grateful that Pat was always there for me when I needed someone to talk with.

Cancer, as we all know, can be an isolating disease for the patient; but unless you have been through it, you may not appreciate that being the supporting partner of a cancer patient can be a lonely path. This path can be made even more lonely if you believe against all the medical odds that the person you are supporting can and will get well.

The third woman whom words could not do justice to was Norma. I shall be ever grateful to her for the generosity of wisdom she so openly shared with me. She supports me still to this day. Her strength even from a distance flowed throughout our healing journey and supported me during the most difficult times of Ian's illness—especially in the early days.

These special women all lent me courage during my different stages of need and I feel I could not have made the journey without them. This experience provided me with a profound understanding of the power of the feminine nature to support, nurture and to provide warmth and wise counsel when required.

Back in the early days of Ian's cancer, with meditation and our new lifestyle, we were going well. After three months of this new approach, tumours that had been previously growing at an alarming rate defied all predictions. They barely increased in size! It was at this point, however, that we experienced a major setback. Ian's pain increased dramatically to a point where meditation could no longer manage it. This, combined with the apparent movement of an enlarged lymph node that had become a bony secondary, resulted in an obstructed ureter and severe kidney problems. Palliative radiotherapy was not effective for the pain and we were fast running out of options. An injection of a natural mistletoe extract brought some relief. So, despite the setback and the pain, at this point we married. Medically it was expected that Ian would live only for a few weeks, but we had other ideas!

Maintaining an undaunting faith in working through the illness, we focused our energies on solutions and possibility thinking. We applied whatever we felt would help Ian's situation but even so there were many highs and lows that we encountered and dealt with on a regular basis. With commitment and zeal we actively continued with our mainstay approaches of nutrition and meditation throughout the years and two and a half years later, in July 1978, Ian was declared cancer free.

It had been a lengthy but rewarding journey back to health.

I too had lived through an extraordinary experience, having been a supporting partner to a cancer patient who journeyed to the edge of life and who survived and thrived despite travelling an often rocky road. The fellow travellers we met along the way who shared their stories, their lives and sometimes even their homes with us, had a lasting impact on us both.

In 1981 we began actively working with cancer patients, founding Australia's first self help cancer support group. This group has evolved into The Gawler Foundation, an international cancer support centre staffed by 33 people and situated in the hills of the picturesque Yarra Valley in Victoria. This residential centre provides active support, education, stress management and meditation training for cancer patients and their families.

A Diploma of Herbal Medicine which I completed with Dorothy Hall has been an added impulse to my work. Dorothy is another of the women of substance who have appeared in my life at times of need. Her comprehensive course, which can best be described as Wholistic Herbalism, had a major impact on me. Much of the healing wisdom that Dorothy was teaching we had applied during the time of Ian's illness and it has been wonderful to be able to incorporate and integrate it into The Foundation's programs.

Working with large groups of people affected by cancer has been a unique opportunity and a profound learning experience. While I regard each patient as an individual and have a dislike for rash generalisations, experience has shown that there has been no avoiding the powerful emergence of common issues and traits among people with cancer. This applies particularly when we consider women with breast cancer as a group.

In relation to stress responses and coping strategies, the patterns we observed in our people correlated with Ainslie Meares' thoughts on the underlying causes of cancer. Prolonged and unresolved stress seemed to be an obvious life pattern in these people. Coupled with this there was usually a major change in life circumstances which appeared to act as the trigger mechanism for the onset of ill health. If one takes the time to listen to the life story of a cancer patient, rather than just concentrating on what is medically wrong with them, a whole new area opens up in understanding the nature of the illness. On a time basis it would be very difficult to do this individually and this is where group work excels. In an atmosphere of support and safety and with the common bond of illness as the carte blanche for sharing and expression, the stories of how people have lived and coped with their lives are both moving and telling.

For women with breast cancer, an effective support group can be a vital link in the progression from stifled silence towards a life of ease where open communication can more readily be expressed and shared. Identifying these patterns, stresses and emotional issues leads to a recognition of the need to encourage more community and social support in the area of illness. Also this applies directly to the prevention of disease, its management and the promotion of healthy lifestyles throughout the community.

It is in the spirit of sharing the experiences and learning of others, that this book is offered.

So why "WOMEN OF SILENCE?"

Women with breast cancer often appear to have developed a way of coping that involves the "bottling up" or withholding of emotional energy of some kind. Usually this emotional energy centres around painful experiences which these women have felt personally incapable of resolving effectively. So, silence instead of expression. This silence is an in-built method of embalming a woman's wounds for reasons of immediate survival and life preservation. Often withholding is the only means of maintaining oneself through crisis. But at some point there needs to be a discharge, a letting go of the event, otherwise its memory will linger on in both the mind and the body. This can lead to an insidious and subtle unease which if unattended, builds up, crisis after crisis, year after year.

Often women have reported to me that this contained emotional energy seems to have quite a specific feeling and a place where it is stored within their being. The feeling they describe as a void. This void feels like an emptiness—an unresolved emptiness. It is a feeling—a space that contains the sense of what is missing and unfulfilled in their life. This feeling of emptiness has a physical location. Asked where it is, most women with breast cancer almost wistfully, invariably gently, tenderly, touch the area over the middle of their chest, or a little lower over their solar plexus.

Most women with breast cancer I have discussed this with immediately recognise this place, the place of the void. Just as quickly, they will say it had been so hard to talk of it, to describe it or share it with anyone else. For many of these women this place had in fact an almost fourth dimensional quality. It went with a feeling of being removed from their customary sense of reality, a feeling of being somehow outside of themselves. Like a portion of them was existing in another dimension—this "fourth" dimension.

Another term I use for this is the inner vessel of the feminine. For this is a place wherein women can seal their silence, seal their pain. With this vessel sealed, the pain contained, coping becomes possible, life can go on—at least on the surface. But the "void" remains—on the inside.

This inner pain and its containment is a feeling common to many women. Having their experience devalued or not even recognised can add to personal frustration and lead to inner suffering. It is this suffering which in turn leads further into the "void."

For many men this will come as useful information. For I believe that many males have quite a different experience and it is my observation, from personal and clinical experience, that very few men come to know how it is for women. Perhaps this relates to what I notice in many men. It seems that their mode of feeling may have a different mechanism of expression compared with many women's modes of feeling. For men, their feeling mode often involves a sense of a deep inner grief. When this inner grief is denied expression, as it often is, it results in a sense of "numbness" to life. This has been described to me many times by men as a feeling of containment rather than a feeling of a void. This numbness or containment dulls the pain allowing men to "soldier on." Again it may be a useful survival mechanism, yet it numbs feelings and prohibits the ability to feel what their partner might be going through.

Although men may be supportive in many ways, and usually this is by doing and filling practical roles, a woman may find that to share her feelings and to have those feelings understood at a gut level may be too much to ask or expect. Sharing feelings then can become a frustration that can make for very dramatic dynamics between men and their wives who are going through breast cancer. Hopefully, reading this book will give men a direct insight into more of what it is to be a woman with breast cancer, and enable them to provide more caring and effective support for their women.

Another key and challenging issue in my work with women with breast cancer has been the observation that a majority of them appear to be calm and passive people in their personality type. But beneath this layer of coping, I have often found that their calmness masks the "void," and that their silence is one of despair and a feeling of hopelessness. Emotions of repressed anger, resentment, unhappiness and discontent are veiled by a passive silence. This silence will produce major hurt and it is also my experience that women with breast cancer can identify readily with this silence.

Yet happily there is another type and quality of silence. Importantly this other silence holds the possibility to heal us.

For there is a creative silence, a nourishing silence, that is the silence of inner peace, the silence of quiet contentment, safe assuredness, limitless potential and joyful expression.

In my view, my experience, real healing can only take place when there is a conscious transition from the state of "bottled up," emotionally distressed silence, to the state of open communication and expression, the state of inner nourishing silence and its product, **PEACE OF MIND.**

I believe that good communication and expression are essential for bringing about the processes that lead towards healing. When we carry too much emotional baggage it is very difficult to experience true peace of mind. However, if expression can be activated along with the will to live and the will to heal, the process of meditation can then be used and developed into a very deep and profound experience of this inner nourishing silence. This type of silence can well be described as the silence of sacred solitude. In these quiet moments of sacred silence, when we experience the stillness of meditation in the gap between thoughts; we are given a glimpse of the possibilities. In that space we have the opportunity to experience our truth—who we really are.

This is where emotional healing is to be found. This experience is like a journey; a journey which offers the very real prospect of being able to live life fully, to realise your goals and to evolve through and beyond the cancer experience.

Such a journey is unique for each woman. Although the physical disease may seem similar in all women, due to different life circumstances, every woman's path to recovery will be uniquely hers.

My hope is that the experience of other women who have travelled that path and shared it with me, combined in this book with my own insight, will help more women to journey with peace and confidence to a land of better health.

Further Recommended Reading:

1. *You Can Conquer Cancer,* by Ian Gawler (Hill of Content Publishing, Melbourne, Australia,)

Chapter Two

Discovering the "Wounds"

Over the years I have spoken with many women affected by breast cancer. From the earliest days I noticed a common fact—so many of these women told stories of extraordinary life experiences. Commonly, they had faced many traumas and hurdles in their lives, yet somehow they managed to adopt coping skills that enabled them to push on and survive. They all displayed a character of great inner strength born of prolonged coping. However, commonly this coping mechanism had come unstuck. It seemed for so many that within their history, a life changing event, an event of insurmountable magnitude had occurred 18 months to two years prior to diagnosis. This seemed to be the proverbial "straw that broke the camel's back," as this event invariably targeted the one vulnerable area in a woman who was otherwise a resilient coper.

These insurmountable issues they describe run the full gamut of human experiences. They include divorce, grief, redundancy, betrayal, bankruptcy, and other similar significant issues. These are not the 'small change' events of life and they seem to have an ability to shock the individual woman to her very marrow. It seems that the vulnerability of women who develop breast cancer lies in the way they attempt to cope with major emotional trauma.

From this original observation, two further streams of thought began to develop. The first was that the different groups or types of cancer patients seemed to have common threads in the fabric of their life story that were specific for that cancer type. It was always noticeable in our groups how those people with the same cancers immediately bonded to each other, not only because of the similarity in illness, but more often it seemed as a consequence of the personal rapport that comes with similarities in personality and nature. While the women with breast cancer were frequently dealing with issues centred around relationship and nurturing, the bowel cancer patients often recognised a combination of diet and prolonged stress as key issues, while brain tumour patients were often aware of mental overloading and mounting pressure in their lives prior to diagnosis.

For example, Virginia was a woman dealing with primary breast cancer. After a lumpectomy and partial reconstruction she sought the support services that our Foundation had to offer. Within the support group, Virginia shared the significant events of recent years that she felt had something to do with her cancer situation.

I have been amazed by the number of women, like Virginia, who of their own volition volunteer the connection between what is going on in their lives and their illness. They also often volunteer in either an embarrassed or matter of fact manner that they did not bother mentioning anything about their personal problems to their doctor for reasons of fear of ridicule or because of the risk of being ignored.

Virginia's life story had a huge impact on the group and there was not a dry eye in the house when she had finished. After having had great difficulty conceiving a child which put enormous pressures on her relationship, Virginia became pregnant and miscarried at 4 months. This traumatic episode occurred twice more! The grief of these experiences was more than she could bear, resulting in her becoming very withdrawn from friends and life in general. She had just discovered that she was pregnant again prior to the diagnosis of her breast lump. As chemotherapy was recommended, and pregnancy viewed as dangerous for a woman with breast cancer, the pregnancy was terminated. Also, Virginia was told that it would be likely that treatment would render future pregnancies impossible. Stories like this are not uncommon in women dealing with breast cancer.

The story of George on the other hand, highlights the different issues in his life. A man of European origin, George had come to Australia and settled with his wife in a small country town where they successfully started a small business. They led a very stressful life, and, as a consequence, his wife Gerta developed chronically high blood pressure and heart problems. Gerta had to retire from the business, leaving George with massive amounts of work to cope with on his own. Realising the work load was beyond him, he hired a partner who ultimately betrayed George's confidence, resulting in the business being declared insolvent. Shortly after, George had a car accident which resulted in even more pressure on an already overloaded financial status. George developed cancer of the sigmoid colon within one year and at the time of diagnosis small secondary tumours were found in the liver. Surgery removed the bowel tumour, but the liver secondaries were not operable. With new information from the cancer support group on board, they began a journey of healing. Together they began to learn about relaxation and stress management and about the role of nutrition. The latter turned out to be the most difficult for George who had left his homeland to live a life that could buy all the wonderful refined foods that were a part of the western lifestyle! He was not impressed with being asked to go back to the unrefined diet of a Polish peasant!

The third example is that of a man called David, who developed a brain tumour. As a committed school teacher he worked 80 hours per week on a regular basis and as well pursued a myriad of hobbies. Sailing was his favourite pastime, but he was so busy, his yacht sat idly by in his back yard waiting for a sailor that never came. A divorce which led to a total separation from his family eventually drove David even harder into what he described as a workaholic state. Eighteen months after the divorce David had a total breakdown and was found to have a large tumour in his brain.

He left work and read as much as he could about what options he had available, as the medical ones were not in his favour. Surgery was not recommended and he refused any other treatment. He now faced life with an understanding that made him feel reconnected to the magic he had lost. He learned to meditate and manage daily stress and began to eat a nutrient dense diet. David survives today, maintaining good health, despite 7 years ago having a prognosis of two years to live.

Inevitably, cancer patients will have a story to tell that is worth listening to! It was noticeable in our support groups, that when people spoke of their lives and their cancers, other patients in the room would begin to nod knowingly as they identified how their own story aligned with those dealing with the same cancer. This is how my views about the nature and origins of breast cancer developed and in the following chapters, I will share more of what I have learned whilst walking on life's path.

But, before we move any further in looking into the origins and causative factors in cancer, I would like to share the second thread which emerged. This I found to be quite exciting and it has provided me which much hope and impetus. Independently, Ian and I had observed that there was a cancer personality type. Other researchers all over the world were identifying the same personality traits. While the issue was contentious and was debated in scientific and medical circles, it was so obvious in our groups, that we knew it had to be of great importance. But then came the wonderful realisation. The more I worked with people affected by cancer, the more I realised that the cancer personality also had its polar opposite, **the survivor personality.**

The seemingly destructive cancer personality and the creative survivor personality were cohabiting side by side within a cancer patient's psyche. The ability to switch off the passion for living message could be transformed into the ability to positively utilise the skills of resilient coping and switch on the survivor message. The strength that ultimately harmed you could be converted into a different strength that could heal you.

Change for some is viewed as unfamiliar territory, rather than a potential that lives within us—all the time. This is one of the valuable lessons I have learned from women with breast cancer. Understanding your strengths provides you with empowerment to translate one type of strength into another. This is how the strength that women had used to withhold emotional energy and which is often a part of the pattern of their disease, can be reframed, then transformed into strengths which have enormous healing potential.

With the inner strength these women developed as they struggled to withhold emotional trauma, there came a related passivity. This passivity appeared to mask the inner turmoil that was felt at many times but not expressed. However, I discovered that many of the women with breast cancer that I was listening to were not passive people by nature, but rather had adopted passiveness as a defence mechanism in order to survive. These women often came to say that the passive silence was developed with a view to keeping the peace. Using this strategy women become more compliant to the wishes of those around them and this was usually demonstrated by a lack of the ability to say "NO!" These women, operating under great emotional pressure in their attempts to survive, learned to become "silent copers."

Joyce's Story—Learning to say No

"Cancer has been my teacher and I have been a slow learner. But what I have learnt is that there is so much help out there to tap into if your are prepared to reach out. Simply try each path that opens up to you until you find the right one for you, that is the ones that touch you deeply.

"I had the first malignant carcinoma in my right breast in1986. After a radical mastectomy my lymph glands were clear and it had been analysed as a primary cancer. My surgeon felt he had "got it all" and the prognosis was very good indeed. I recovered well and got back into the "busy-ness" of life again, feeling I had been "lucky." Exactly two years later in 1988 I had visited my surgeon for a check-up and he was surprised to find another lump in the remaining breast. He arranged a mammogram and an ultrasound there and then, and as he had just had a patient cancel an operation the following morning, he offered to slot me into that time if I would like to take it. So after a phone call to my husband I proceeded straight to the hospital. My husband was shocked, duly arrived and agreed it was better to get it over without delay.

"My surgeon followed the same procedure as the first time, that is removing the lump and having pathology on it whilst I was anaesthetised, and, as it was malignant, removing the whole breast and lymph glands. It was another primary cancer and oestrogen positive, whereas the first one was progesterone positive, but again my lymph glands were clear and so I felt incredibly "lucky" as he had "got it all." My surgeon and I both said, it can't happen again! It was true enough, with the loss of both breasts and very much a Pollyanna attitude.

"I decided as I went to acquire my second prosthesis, I could now be flexible and I chose to come down a size in bust measurement. It took me longer to recover the second time and I had to have my large keloid scar cut and redone as it was painful and waking me up at night. I had six radiation treatments to slow down the healing of the scar and I eventually started to feel comfortable once more.

"Then in May 1991 my world fell apart and was shattered with the result of my bone scan that I had because of pain in my left ribs. The original pain was a red herring and not related to bone cancer, but it fortunately enabled early detection of the twelve secondary tumours peppered through my bone in the neck, spine, clavicle, arm, ribs, hips and leg. The medical treatment prescribed was Nolvadex-D (Tamoxifen), a hormonal treatment taken orally. I must say at this point that I consider myself fortunate in having the wonderful doctors I have. My wonderful GP over 20 years helped me with acupuncture and encouragement.

"Likewise my surgeon of over 15 years, whom I have utmost faith in, helped and encouraged me. So, knowing I had the best medical help available, I knew that I must reach out and tap into that best of self-help programs that spoke to me. We attended a residential program at The Gawler Foundation and also a program run by Petrea King in Sydney. What an experience and journey lay ahead. I had no idea it could be so rewarding, fulfilling and exciting. At that point I decided that I was a very inhospitable host to this cancer invading my body and life and as I was rapidly running out of options, decided to give it my undivided attention.

"I then had my December scan and it was all clear of any active cancer. Truly a miracle! So now there is no way we would change our new lifestyle as it is far better than life before cancer. The whole experience has taught us how very precious life is and never to take it for granted. We live in the moment and enjoy each day. Love is the key and I have so much surrounding me from my family and wonderful friends. My wonderful husband has always remained positive and we share so much more than ever before.

"I believe that another important part of my healing is that I have learnt to say "NO." So I continue to set more realistic goals and look forward to the next half of my life with hope and joy. I no longer am afraid of cancer. I am certainly more in touch with my higher self and higher power.

"I have a PEACE OF MIND now that is a priceless gift and my heart is full of gratitude."

Footnote: Joyce remains well to this day.

(Joyce's story is reproduced in full in *Patient Profiles,* an inspiring booklet produced by The Gawler Foundation).

Chapter Three

Emotional Patterns of Breast Cancer

It takes a great deal of inner energy and strength to withhold, internalize or contain what are really natural emotional responses to life. When we are hurt, we cry. When we are happy, we smile and laugh. When we are deeply saddened we grieve. Ideally we would be able to feel comfortable expressing those feelings rather that being bound to "keep a stiff upper lip" and soldier on. For repressing emotions can lead to a disturbing sense that we are not living true to ourselves; while it can lead to those around us believing that we can cope, when in reality we cannot.

I find the symbolism of language to be quite fascinating in situations where emotional expression may be an issue. For example, in cancer detection, the word "screening" is used. A mammogram for instance is used to screen you. The word screen, implies that there is something hidden that the screen test has to find. My suggestion is that we also need to "screen" our emotions to discover what is hidden in issues that may be related to breast cancer. What "knots" may be found in our psyche, or even deeper still, what "knots" may be hidden in our souls? Who knows, one day such tests may be available!

Fatigue

One of the first early warning signs of breast cancer can be extreme fatigue that is not relieved by sleep or rest. This tiredness shows us that the chronic build-up of stress held in the mind is being mirrored in the body. We feel this as fatigue. As the build-up of stress in our inner and outer world becomes greater, there is often an impending sense of doom and powerlessness to do anything about it.

All too often women, being the carers and nurturers, easily give and give of themselves. This giving may be just in relationship to her family; it may be in relation to giving her all to work; it may even be a combination of all this and more!

It may be that a woman gives 150% of herself to her career and then becomes tired, jaded and unhappy with how her life has become. Another example might be a busy executive who is also a mother—torn between the need to be the perfect mother and to be perfectly available for her career. Knowing how impossible all this is, and all the time feeling that her attempts to nurture her job, her husband and children are just not working. Trying hard to meet all the demands, she silently keeps going, feeling it is all just too much. Fatigue is an obvious consequence of all this.

Distorted Nurturing, Twisted Emotions

Women easily develop a tendency to give of themselves by overnurturing others and undernurturing themselves in the giving of love. What causes this to happen, what is behind it all, is so often emotionally based. For example, with single women, the breakdown of a significant relationship that had been cherished and nurtured could be a key stress factor in the pattern of their breast cancer development. The detail of these traumatic experiences may be different for different people, but the pattern is so familiar. The way I know that makes sense of this is to listen to people's stories.

The following examples of life patterns are quite typical of how many women describe what their life was like before they developed breast cancer, of how their fatigue developed, and how it affected them.

Firstly women with breast cancer often notice that one positive benefit of having given of themselves and of being there for everyone all the time was that "approval" came in large doses. This "giving of self" so often explains why women with breast cancer are thought of as being "nice" people. Of course they are "nice"—they are always helpful, always there. The first to be at the school fete at 6a.m. so that others do not have to get there so early. The women who also probably stayed up the night before baking scones, making jam and hemming a party dress for a favourite daughter. Breast cancer patients can be terrific mums, but they may sacrifice their energy to their own detriment!

Now some women can be perfectly contented, happy and healthy, giving freely of themselves. It is a fact that for some women selfless service is an uncomplicated joy. But the key here is what drives that service; and how the woman nurtures herself. For if a woman has totally devoted her life to her family and she has never considered herself as an individual who also needs nurturing, she becomes very vulnerable. It is bound to happen one day that she will be left with no one to give out to. With no experience of giving to herself, faced with a lack of nurturing from both the inside and the outside, the sudden awareness of the void will become evident. The baby birds have flown the nest, the nest is empty and suddenly so is life. I have seen this pattern in many women past the age of 40. It is as if their reason to be is no longer there.

Alternatively, a woman may be tirelessly giving out to her family and all goes well for a few years. Children grow, husbands get busy and people forget to notice what is being done for them. Now the "joy" of doing becomes the "resentment" of doing. The whole picture begins to take a downhill slide. Sadly, I recently met a woman in this situation who was dealing with very advanced secondary breast cancer, and who, despite loving her family, resented everything about her life with them. She was very "stuck" in this pattern and was so "silent" that she was almost paralysed to communicate at all. Trapped as she was, trapped in an endless cycle of resentment, suffering and self pity from which it seemed no one could retrieve her, she did confide in me saying that she just wanted to go. She was tired of living. She died two weeks later.

Take heed—fatigue may be an early warning worth listening to. On a prevention basis, taking regular time out for yourself could be life saving. Fatigue, if unattended to in a woman who leads an active life, can develop into the next stage of the pattern which is the requirement of more and more willpower to keep the body going.

In this scenario, no matter how exhausted a woman really feels, still there is the silence; and the tired body meekly follows along underneath a wilful and strong head. After all, this woman knows a lot about stress, a lot about coping, it has always been her way. So, no matter how exhausted she is, this **dependable** woman is always there. But the inner woman begins to crave solitude. Finally she can no longer ignore the signals from within. She starts to get a sense of what is missing in her life—time for herself. With the lack of personal space the inner tension begins to mount and finally she is confronted with the fact that she is:

... living a lifestyle out of control,
Too much held in too often has taken its toll.

Feeling powerless to act, feeling a sense of hopelessness to change, the silence becomes sealed deep within. Paradoxically, however, the void is filled. It is filled with emotional, physical and spiritual pain that causes unrelenting ill ease!

Again this feeling of impending doom is talked about by women who have been through the breast cancer experience. Despite instincts that are wounded, bodies that are tired and spirits that are low, it is not until diagnosis time that they have a reason to stop. Now their inner life has demanded it.

Linda's Story

Linda discovered a breast lump which was confirmed to be cancerous in 1982. At that time she refused a mastectomy and just had the lump removed. This was followed with 30 days of radiotherapy. At the time Linda had just returned from a period of living in the U.S.

"I had worked as a receptionist/assistant in a Holistic medical clinic there and had seen many people getting well. My marriage had collapsed in America and when I came back to Australia, deep inside, I really wanted to die. I felt I couldn't do it directly to myself, however the cancer decided to try to do it for me. However, once I had the surgery and began radiation, I was getting pretty cross with myself for wanting to die—just because someone else didn't think I was good enough! So I began using meditation, active visualisation and vitamin and mineral supplements. Because I only had the lump out, I had a heavy treatment schedule. Yet, despite the warnings of pain and other side effects, I was the only one of the ten ladies who went through with me that had no problems.

"For the first time, this caused me to begin to feel that I could **have some power over my own life.** That was really exciting! Since then however, there have been some lapses in faith. Eighteen months after the surgery, in 1984, a nodule appeared in my thyroid. I requested one month to work on it and sure enough it decreased. Now, if I get stressed, up it comes. I intensify the efforts, regain the balance, down it goes. I seem able to control it.

"Through all this, I came to know that those who faced death and saw it as a new beginning could let go and have a good death. That has helped me a lot. You know my mother often told me as a child that she wanted to die. **I picked it up** and have had trouble getting over it fully and I know that for years it interfered with me maintaining the **joy of life.** It has been a strong emotional habit to break. Now I pray a lot, I could not have made it without prayer. At the moment I want to work on myself. I am in a conventional job and my husband is back in my life. I am learning a lot about male/female relationships.

"**I believe I got cancer in the breast because I was not nurturing myself.** When my children were young I used to have these horrible nightmares. I was suckling this thin wretched whimpering child who had a smelly nappy on and appeared so uncared for. I could never understand it, as **I gave everything I had to my children.** Only recently when I was sick did I realise that the child was **myself!**

"Now I don't flagellate myself. **I can accept myself** and where I am at. I continue to meditate and get closer to my spiritual self. I aim to change slowly. I have good days and bad ones, but mostly good. Cancer has pointed me in the right spiritual direction. I have learnt how the mind does control the body. The material and worldly things have become less important, although I still love to dress up. I have met and shared with so many people that I have a better perspective now. I also believe that death as a conscious experience is very important—especially if it is a part of living."

It seems that the need to take control of one's life when dealing with breast cancer comes up time and time again. In the process of healing this is a necessity according to those who have healed. We lose control in so many ways, so easily and so often for reasons that may have apparently noble causes. Loss of control, however, ultimately leads to a loss of spirit or power.

Some define healing as bringing your spirit home, or taking your power back consciously and methodically from all the people to whom you have given it away. This taking control of one's life again goes hand in hand with taking responsibility for yourself and for your life. It is a huge step to take. However, not only is this an important step in the realm of self help approaches in healing; but having control over what happens to you within the boundaries of your medical treatment can really make a difference to the outcome. In order to survive, you may have to speak up, ask questions and assert yourself when necessary. Remember, it is your body and it will be you who has to live with the consequences of whatever approach you choose.

Further Recommended Reading:

1. *Cancer as a Turning Point,* Lawrence Le Shan, Ph.D. (Pub. by Plume.)
2. *The Heroic Path,* by Angela Passidomo Trafford (Pub. by Blue Dolphin.)

Chapter Four

Breast Cancer, How and Why

When we hold our silence, withhold our feelings, withhold our love, withhold the nurturing of ourselves, we stifle our passion, our *joie de vivre*. The ability to hold silence and adopt a passive approach that is not a part of a women's natural character is equivalent to putting a tight lid on a saucepan that is trying to boil over.

A woman in a recent group program called Sally, shared this story with us. As a woman currently dealing with breast cancer, she told of how her family had been concerned for her health before her diagnosis. For a long time she was always stressed, feisty and became angry easily. Her family were also having trouble coping with her erratic behaviour. So, without dealing with the stress problems, Sally tried to adopt a new way of coping and, in her words, "bit her tongue" when she wanted to display her feistiness. However, the result was that Sally went about her daily business feeling like an unexploded volcano! She was not used to living her life to please other people and after all, according to Sally, she had plenty of things in her life to be fiery about! Within a year, Sally began to experience an extreme fatigue and lethargy. A general checkup with her G.P. resulted in a breast lump being detected and when biopsied, it was found to be malignant. A large portion of breast was removed. She took the opportunity in one of our groups to use her keen and feisty wit. She said to her husband sitting next to her "Well, see where all this got me. Thank God I've got a good excuse now to go back to being my old self again!"

Emotional energy by its very nature is a dynamic energy. As emotion is felt, it finds its expression in the outer world, with what we experience as happiness, joy, excitement, love, grief, anger, resentment, rage and so on. My definition of depression is the absolute non-movement of emotion, characterized by a blankness of expression or feeling. However, as I see it, at least true depression is obvious if the person is experiencing it.

But, what if that person felt depressed, dis-spirited and tried to pretend that all in life was sunny and wonderful? I ask where would the depression go? It would still be there. It would still be housed in the mind, the psyche and the body, but it would be consciously blocked from finding outer expression.

The following exercise may help to clarify this. Close your eyes for a moment and think of a time when you experienced spontaneous happiness in your life. Maybe it was a surprise or good news of some kind. As you think about that time, consciously go through the memories, imagine the scene, the tastes, smells, sounds and sensations and notice how these memories have feelings associated with them. Experience those feelings for a few moments; notice the affects of the memories and then open your eyes. If you re-experienced a truly happy and joyful event, you will notice a sense of good feeling in the body. Your immune system is likely to have responded in a positive way; and also maybe now you also have a sense of the animated movement of emotional energy.

But what happens if we hold in emotional energy? Interestingly, as we discussed already, it is the more negative emotions that we are likely to hold on to, and they are the ones that literally "eat holes" in us. It seems, however, that we are not so likely to do it with the positive emotions in life. Sometimes we might have suppressed positive feelings if we had parents who said "Wipe that smile off your face right now!" But that was usually short lived and we had a good laugh as soon as they were out of sight!

Where withholding positive emotions can be a significant problem, is where they are held for fear of these emotions not being accepted by the people we love. Women with breast cancer often demonstrate this and it can take many different forms of expression. One of the symptoms of this is women's tendency to give out care and love to everyone else around, while at the same time finding difficulty in accepting the love that is being given to them. At the root of this problem is an inability to give love to themselves—to be self nurturing. This, in my experience revolves around a chronic lack of self esteem, or self worth. Often there is a sense of these emotions or even the woman herself being devalued.Many of my breast cancer patients have strongly identified with this aspect in their own experience.

This pattern of emotional suppression or denial can and often does lead on to extreme fatigue. This is what the women describe when they say they are feeling "sick at heart." So, with their "battery flat," women often have to drive on, utilising sheer willpower, masking their inner fatigue in order to survive. Often these women have great difficulty asking for help, because they are the people that everyone has learned to rely upon and as a result they have no ability to say "no." They could not possibly let people down!

No one lives in a vacuum in this world, and stress generated from one's outer life experience adds to the load. The internal stress from withholding and the external stress of living means that somewhere, somehow, something has to give. It is usually these women's health that pays the price, presenting them with a definite ultimatum for change and transformation—breast cancer.

The following story of Dallas' brush with breast cancer back in December 1983, highlights some of the above points. The way she tells her story reflects her true nature now, which she demonstrates with good humour and verve!

Dallas' Story

A biopsy of a breast lump in December 1983 was treated with great suspicion by Dallas' doctor, although it was three days before the positive diagnosis of cancer was confirmed. According to Dallas:

"The initial reaction was panic. Really, I felt like I was looking possible death in the eyeball. I thought of the family particularly, and how they would cope. **I didn't cry during the day and no one knew or picked it up.** The nights were the worst. Every so often I would get this feeling of blind panic. After the three days I had sorted it out and prepared myself. Surgery was recommended immediately, but I wanted to make sure it had not spread and insisted on scans. These were clear, but after the surgery it was found that two lymph nodes were affected.

"The surgeon described the cancer as a "virulent little bastard!" and wanted me to have chemo. I took hours of convincing as I was concerned about depressing my immune system. The doctor convinced me I had no other choice, so I began a 12 month course.

"It was hell. The worst year of my life. I managed to keep working, just taking 5 days off each month. But it was not just how sick it left me feeling, but the other things with the body. I guess I do resent it in many ways, because of the changes that took place, that I think I am stuck with. With the premature menopause, the hot flushes, the loss of taste and smell and the hypersensitivity to some things. Aerosol sprays still nearly make me throw up. I guess I kept going for the children mostly. At first all the family were keen for me to have it, but after 3 months they wanted me to stop. I guess I felt I had committed myself and told myself it was going to work, so I stuck with it. Hardest bloody 12 months of my life!

"However, it was really quite humbling through all this to become aware of the incredible number of people who were so caring. It made me more aware of what makes the world go around."

Twelve months of chemotherapy completed, Dallas then discovered that she had cervical dysplasia.

"I overheard it actually at the doctors. It seems they didn't tell me at the first sign—3 months earlier, as they didn't want to worry me! At the second test, the area affected was clearly visible. It was then that I thought that I had to do something for myself. I had always believed in the power of the mind, but was unsure of how to use it, so, I began talking to this area of my body and pretty simply told the problem to go away. Attending a 10 day residential program with the Gawlers gave me the tools to work with, although by that time the dysplasia had cleared anyway. My main focus though was to stay well from then on.

"If I get tired now, I know I get problems. It's very important to keep yourself on an even keel. I do that with meditation, diet and attitude. The meditation helps with the kids too. After a good session in the morning, even a little monster can't touch me, try as they might!

"Cancer has brought a new perspective to my life. In the long term it has led to a sorting out of priorities. I now appreciate people more and see things through different eyes. I appreciate the country even more, take time to look at something—a simple thing that is really beautiful. It's a heightening of awareness. Things that I was vaguely aware of before, took for granted in fact, are now so wonderful.

"Relationships have changed a bit. I am less inclined to let others organise my time for me now. I am much more aware of the value of time and my need to control it. And, I am probably less tolerant of crap—you know, from other people. I either avoid it or I am more direct; say what I think and express my opinion more. I am not so prepared to compromise myself, and put up with it."

"Well, I don't get angry, okay? I mean I have a tendency to internalize. I can't express anger. That's one of the problems I have.

I - I grow a tumour instead."

(Isaac Davis in *Manhattan* by Woody Allen and Marshall Brickman)

Why Do People React in this Way?

As a product of our experience and perceptions of early life we may be pre-programmed to internalize feelings that otherwise we would be better off releasing. During the difficult and traumatic times of our lives we learn to cope in particular ways. These ways may be a great help to us in the future, or they may not, depending on who we are as individuals and whether the adopted style of coping allows us to live true to our nature.

It seems there is little doubt that the environment which we grew up and developed in, including the influence of parents and other people, has quite an influence on our emotional responses and our ability to express our emotions. Clearly as children, we often adopt subconsciously, or even consciously, attitudes and behaviours of those close to us. Maybe your husband has said to you in a heated moment:

"You're getting more like your mother every day. That's what she would have said!..."

And the same can be said of wives to husbands as well: *"You know, you are just like your father. Can't you just feel a little more?..."*

This pattern of conditioned learning at a young age is termed "premature cognitive commitment," which basically means that we make a commitment to a certain way of learning how to be, at an early age. This "setting" of responses is often the reason why many people find great difficulty accepting and activating change in their lives. Their "commitment" to follow a certain way of behaving in the world is so strong, so embedded, that it has become part of their life's belief system.

To clarify this mechanism, I will describe a simple behavioural experiment with flies! If you place a number of flies in a jar covered with wire they will happily fly around and around perceiving that the jar is "their space." Eventually, when the wire is removed, the flies have an obvious escape route. However, although we have given them the opportunity to fly out and away, the majority of them will stay within the confines of the jar! They have made a behavioural "commitment" that the jar is where they are to stay. Only one or two "pioneer" flies will leave the jar and escape!

I cannot help but see the analogy between this simple experiment and my work with cancer patients (without appearing insulting and comparing them to flies!) However, the "pioneer" flies symbolize the patients who recognise another way, a way through and out of cancer and do not fulfil their commitment to stay "stuck" in the confines of what "should" happen to them! Like Dallas in our story—she knew there had to be another way and that she needed to learn to help her self.

So, our perceptions, the way we view the world and the way we behave, are all influenced by these early experiences. In any traumatic situation or challenge, we **clearly do the best we can at the time.** In considering all of this **be gentle with yourself**. Some of the ways we have used to cope in the past, we may not feel so good about now. But remember back to that time. What else did we know? What else could we have done? At least we can **congratulate ourselves for making it through at all.** We may be a little worn around the edges, but we are still here!

Obviously some of our patterns of behaviour have been quite effective, perhaps even essential in helping us through a particular life crises. Perhaps, for example, the stifled silence was the only way we thought we could keep the peace or endure a tragedy and keep going. The question is do we still want to keep doing that? (Like the flies in the jar!) Have we now got other options, (The lid is removed from the jar) and **would doing it differently work better for us now?** (The "pioneer" flies find a new way of behaving.)

For some women, their early life history may be more important than for others. This is particularly so for those women who have experienced major personal tragedies, such as sexual abuse, during their lives. This issue needs to be addressed, as so many women with breast cancer, so many women of silence, have shared it with me. It is by nature an emotionally charged subject, but I feel that often it is an essential ingredient in healing the feminine. If it is a part of a woman's emotional history, it needs to be a part of her current healing agenda.

If I had not had so many stories volunteered and shared with intense sincerity over the years, I might have presumed that coincidence was at play here. However, this has been such a common issue, not only for women dealing with breast cancers, but female reproductive cancers of all kinds, that I feel impelled to share it. Please understand this may have been an important issue for some, but clearly not all women with breast cancer.

I have given the following section a great deal of consideration due to its intimate and powerful nature. Choosing to exclude it could leave a cloud of unknowing for the many women who in reality have faced sexual abuse in their lives and who already know or sense that this event has some significance in their illness.

Basically there are three groups of women to whom this issue of sexual abuse applies. Firstly I hope that this discussion may open the door for those women who so far are basically healthy, have experienced sexual abuse in their lives, but feel helpless to resolve it and therefore have been withholding it entirely. I feel this to be an imperative in the area of women's health, for, as a natural health practitioner, I have discovered that the subject of sexual abuse seems to be linked to many chronic female problems such as chronic vaginitis, cervical dysplasia, frigidity, difficulty with periods and a wide variety of other female problems. Usually this is not volunteered by the patient until the second or third visit, when enough relationship had been established to secure trust. Quite often the subject is broached by the statement, "I don't know if this has anything to do with my condition but..."and the story begins with a tone of relief that implies: "At last this is someone I can tell." So, I am convinced that this has to be an area where disease prevention can be really put into action at a community level.

The second group of women is the group who already have been given a diagnosis of cancer, whether it be in the breast or reproductive areas. These women have been very conscious of the fact that sexual abuse was an issue in their lives and when their diagnosis came, often they were not surprised. My experience here too, is that although they were fully aware that this issue had affected them in the past, and was still affecting them in their current life, they had not sought help or spoken about it with anyone. It was only when the illness developed and they joined in with a group, only when they saw and related to other people in similar difficulties, that the "ice was broken." Finally they could speak after years of imposed silence. In private counselling, the problem of prolonged frigidity often comes up in conversation.

I can remember a time during a residential group where a courageous middle aged woman spoke before the group, announcing that she had been a victim of incest. Her husband, also in the room, was extremely shocked and surprised. He had not known. However, he did say that sexual relations had always been difficult for them and now at least it made some sort of sense to him. Fortunately their relationship was rock solid, so together they worked it out. Added to the woman's new found ability not to remain silent, her husband's ability to be a warm and particularly caring and understanding man was exactly what she needed. I am constantly aware of how different people need all kinds of different things in order to heal. This one episode was a key for her. She began responding to chemotherapy after that time and recovered fully.

Finally, to the third and last group. For these women, the problem of sexual abuse has not been obvious. Initially it was not within the grasp of the women's conscious minds. However, they did have an innate awareness of some aspect of their sexual feelings being peculiar and that sexual relationships had always been a difficult area of their life. Most of these women I have come to know quite well and they will still contact me for a chat. It seems that their recovery can be quite a long one and maybe this is due to the fact that their abuse was buried and out of conscious awareness for such a long time.

It was not until my first two patients with repressed abuse problems were in the final stages of dying that they actually spoke of it. This made me aware that maybe their outcomes could have been different. With both these women I had been aware of some sort of enormous pain and my "gut feeling" was that abuse of some kind had taken place. In order to make survival possible, the entire event had been filed away, out of conscious access. However, through the process of meditation and coming to peace with themselves, the fragmented and repressed issues of their lives were dealt with and were shared with their partners just prior to death.

Importantly, however, I do believe that these women, at the end of their lives found healing. Both their partners wrote to me of their experiences with great sensitivity and understanding. They also commented that these open discussions prior to the death of their wives, enabled them to cope better with the grief afterwards.

These days, I refer people to specialist counsellors for guidance if I suspect there may be a problem in this area. So far this has been helpful, but it can take a long time to recover.

Dealing with guilt is usually a problem for all women coping with sexual abuse. As well there may be real problems with their self esteem which is often low. Jenny's story may help to share the significance of this issue in this third group of women.

Jenny's Story

Jenny had endured a long struggle with secondary cancer after an initial mastectomy in 1989. She often experienced a great deal of inner tension and feelings of generally not being at ease with herself. However, she found great solace in reconnecting with her religion. She had been highly passionate about it many years ago, but for some unknown reason had let it slip away out of her life. She was experiencing deep feelings of guilt about many things and found her reconnection with the church a great source of comfort. Over a period of time her spirit and determination to heal was getting stronger and stronger, but her physical condition was becoming weaker. Rarely had I observed such passion to heal in a patient who was so ill for so long.

It took two years before the issue of prolonged sexual abuse in her life was ready to be dealt with. It was Jenny who made this decision to deal with these issues after a skilled G.P. friend of mine realised their existence. This fortunately coincided with a time when she was spiritually able to cope with facing the past and the insidious effects it was having on her life now. Some time later she related to me how she innately knew that the sexual area of her life was badly out of balance because of something really major, but she had no idea what was the cause. I found it interesting that she said the following, "It was as if my body knew, my body remembered what had happened to it, especially when my husband came near me at night. I would go sort of rigid. It was as if my entire reproductive system would go into "shut-down." But my mind knew nothing, no reason. We attended marriage counselling for some time, but it didn't help."

But now Jenny's burden was beginning to lift after re-experiencing the memory of these painful events. Inside was a veritable Pandora's box of abuse. However, she courageously "faced the tiger" and piece by piece, began to restore the fragments of her life into wholeness. The story that she told was of a father with a voracious appetite for sexual activity. Every time her mother was away, which was often, her father would make her appease his needs. He was very fond of groping and handling her breasts and for years afterwards the breast area for her became in her words "not handleable territory."Her experience led her to great guilt, shame and a sense of powerlessness that left her feeling empty and alone, but still she loved and cared for her father enormously. She was "his little princess."And so, at such a young age began the development of another woman of silence.

In order to heal Jenny began the process of forgiving her father. She said that due to her religious feelings, she could now do it, but that actually the hardest part was forgiving herself; learning to let go of the guilt and the shame and the feeling that her illness had been a justified punishment for her actions.

"Ridding myself of my breast didn't rid myself of my problems, but maybe it gave me more time to deal with them," she said.

Jenny feels today as if the weight of the world is off her shoulders. Still she has not lost her sense of humour when she comments, "I guess I've got it off my chest at last!" She is most grateful to the kind and patient doctor who is still helping her through her ordeal." I still have quite a bit of pain from all the bone secondaries, but I believe I'm now healed." Jenny continues her brave struggle for survival.

As difficult as it may be to write about these unpleasant facts of life, I am impelled and encouraged by the women who have felt that for them this was a significant issue to be dealt with. No, the memories are not removed, but the emotional sting, the inner hurt, the inner pain can be dealt with, and, although wounded deeply, as with most wounds that heal—scars form. You are aware of their presence, they are reminders of what you have gone through, but congratulate yourself that you have survived; you have made it through one of the most traumatic issues that could ever be in a woman's life. Now, make the transition from surviving to thriving, speak when you feel ready to, seek the help and wise counsel you need and begin to regain the passion for life that still dwells within.

In conclusion, I will share with you the wise words of a sign that appeared on one of our local churches. This saying reflects Jenny's new philosophy of living:

> *"When trouble overtakes you*
> *Let God take over!"*

Jenny also believes now that the ordeals life presents do not have punishment as their goal, but rather they offer an opportunity for transformation.

Further Recommended Reading:

1. *The Creation of Health,* by C. Norman Shealy, M.D. Ph.D. and Caroline M. Myss, M.A. (Pub. by Stillpoint.)

Chapter Five

Beginning to Reclaim Your "Magic"

Steps towards helping yourself

Making personal changes and transformations can be for like leaping off the precipice into the unknown. This can become even more risky if your health is frail, but it can be the very challenge that can turn obstacles into opportunities.

Remember always—that the only real freedom we have in this life is to choose how we respond to it. People who demonstrate a survivor personality often have had many experiences in their life that have shaped them into the people we are in awe of. They too have come to crossroads in their life, often through means other than illness that have clearly demanded changes. Importantly, survivors realised at that point that they had a choice—a choice of how they would respond. These are the people who made the courageous decision to "face the tiger," and discovered once they had faced it, that it was not nearly so scary, but held something quite wonderful, quite "magical."

For example, they are people who climb mountains in order to reach that special moment of "magic"—the magic of reaching the pinnacle and viewing the world from its highest point.

I had the pleasure of spending some time with the late Sir Edward "Weary" Dunlop a couple of years ago and spent time talking about this issue. His insights about survival and the nature of survivors was, of course, a result of his experience in World War Two as a Doctor in a P.O.W. camp in Burma. One incident we spoke about was when he was found to be insubordinate and was to executed. In fact, this happened many times, and he spoke humbly about his reprieves. He spoke of his fear in the face of his demise, but how he realised that he had a choice about how he responded to the crisis. He had watched the demise of other men in the face of fear when they had lost their centre and saw themselves as doomed. I am not suprised that he was to become a leading cancer surgeon, whose patients adored him. He was able to assist them, not only with their physical problems, but he had an innate understanding of their suffering, and was therefore able, through his presence, to lend them the courage to heal and to reclaim their "magic."

The art of positive survival is innate in us all; we are all born survivors, but some do not take the opportunity to "seize the day," "seize the moments" that are the Godgiven opportunities that can release us from the mould of ordinary existence.

You see, many people incorrectly believe that change will strip them of their identity. But to view this differently, *transformation* may not be taking on anything new, but rather dropping off layers of the old, revealing who and what was there all the time. This then becomes like looking at the world through new eyes. The first step is deciding that you want to do it! Then the possibilities open up and the "magic" can happen.

This "magic" happens when we have a sense of a different dimension in our lives. Many have experienced its power. Remember the first time you fell in love! Healing can be like having a love affair with yourself. After all these years you will have someone quite wonderful and exciting on the inside just waiting for an introduction!

Meditation practise can be reflected into your outer life by sheer radiance of presence and a *joie de vivre* that is a natural consequence. Language is inadequate to describe the beauty of this state, but once you have touched it, you know it's there.

Ainslie Meares often said, "It is like trying to tell someone what a banana tastes like when they have never tasted one!" I have often had the comment from women after they have "touched" that place, that they feel as if they could live or die and "know" that they would be alright. This is because touching the "inner magic" gets us in touch with who we really are. Then we can begin the most intimate relationship with ourselves and it will radiate to all around us.

The first hint of "magic" working in your life on an outer level may manifest itself in the sudden influx of coincidences. This might be termed a state of heightened conscious awareness. For instance, a book may fall from a shelf and when you look down, there before you lies the answer to a problem or question you have been giving serious thought to. A friend may make a comment that provides a significant insight for you, just at the right time. Inspiration is around us in abundance if we can open ourselves to the possibilities.

During Ian's illness we had many times when finances were really stretched and money would be sent anonymously in cash or as bank cheques. Like the birds of the air, we were never without seed.

These little glimpses of the nature of "magic" can lead the way into a deeper level of "ancient magic" that runs so deep, it feels as if it flows in our blood and through to our very souls. For women, this "old magic" comes from the instinctive, intuitive, feminine principle which is now waking up and offering access to a storehouse of wisdom. It probably carries the innate wisdom of all the women who have gone before you; it is like a blueprint of feminine energy.

I once heard a wonderful talk by Jungian analyst Robert Johnson on the Transformations of Life. He stated that a woman who is living true to her nature, never really leaves the hall of wisdom and therefore never needs to search for wisdom in the outside world for it dwells within her all the time. Men on the other hand, he said, need to search for the experience in the outer world in order to be initiated and reconnected to their wisdom. They need to go off on their quests of courage and bravery to find out who they are.

As women enter their hall of wisdom, where the "old magic" lies, it is as if we become in tune or rhythm with the sound and cycles of our hearts and souls. This experience is accessible to all women. It knows no social, ethnic or financial boundary. I have recognised this quality in some of the poorest women in India and throughout many parts of Asia. I have experienced its presence and power in Afro-American women and in our Australian Aboriginal women. These are women of their own power who know how to connect with the "magic," the sacred; that which provides such unique sustenance in a woman's life. Without it, she never feels complete, and if she mistakenly takes the masculine path into the outside world to provide her with sustenance, she will always be feeling hungry and undernourished—and wondering why.

This state of "inner magic" can neither be controlled nor touched by knowledge, reason or rational thinking. It just is. I know I was able to tune in to this level of understanding when Ian was in the midst of his cancer experience and I know the strength I drew from it. It sustained me throughout. Twenty years on, I am still making withdrawals from this endless supply of nourishment. It fuels me to continue on.

With this process in motion, many patients have said to me, "I now know that I can get well. I do not just think it or hope it, I know it! I do not know how, in fact everything modern medicine knows and has to offer says that I am not likely to recover. I can't put words around it. I just know!"

These women were right—they did know and they learned how to heal with zeal—the subject of Part Two of *Women of Silence.*

Further Recommended Reading:

1. *Fire in the Soul,* by Joan Borysenko (Pub. by Warner Books.)

Part Two

"...find the courage to heal
and sing your heart's song..."

Chapter Six

Beginning To Heal With Zeal

You will be aware that in this book so far I have described many aspects of the feminine nature—the female mode of being. I have described how the bottling up of dynamic emotional energy that required expression leads to fatigue and spells danger to a woman's health. All of this is in relation to the feminine way.

So now we need to consider how to initiate healing. The first step in emotional healing is the **acknowledgement** to yourself of how it has been for you. This may simply involve telling your story, thus bringing your life history to conscious awareness. Journal writing can also work extremely well for those who still find the idea of speaking out to either a group or an individual a little daunting. Most people are amazed to read their life story in this type of format. Telling your story has the power to gently tap into memory and therefore shift and bring movement to stuck emotional patterns. Remember to have the courage to allow expression of any emotions that arise naturally during this process of acknowledgement.

The second step is to **recognise that change is required** as the way in which you have coped is no longer appropriate. Consider that so far your life is a product of the past. Simply, are you happy with your life now? What is important for you to change to make it better and to provide a healing environment? It seems that for each woman with breast cancer there are issues that revolve around nurturing and relationship. Choose the key events that you recognise as important, as for each woman they will be different and result from individual life experience. No one can make the changes for you.

The third step is to acknowledge and **have respect for the feelings that you have withheld.** Remembering that they are a part of you, begin the process of gently and respectfully releasing them. I believe this third process to be highly important in the healing process. For women, putting a "lid" of positive thinking principles on top of unrecognised, ignored or unreleased emotions is not being honest with yourself. **Healing requires that we are honest with ourselves.** Allow yourself the luxury to "bottom out" for a day or two. Throughout the entire process of your healing give yourself time out and the luxury of a low energy day every now and then. Some people have a misconception that healing is about being warm and sunny all the time. It is not. It is about being **real, honest and true to yourself.**

Being "sunny" all the time requires a lot of energy and is not really being true to the female mode of feeling either. Just as males and females are different in obvious ways, so are their modes of feeling as different as chalk and cheese. Have you ever noticed how many motivational, mind power, positive thinking books are written by men?

Men have the innate ability to perform, to be sunny and more constant. They are more linear in their nature. Women are lunar—of the moon by nature. Indeed our hormonal cycles are 28 day lunar cycles. What does the moon do? It waxes and wanes. The tides ebb and flow, just like the emotional feeling patterns of a woman's life. This is her natural way. Using the analogy of the moon, when the moon is shining so are we, but remember the moon has a period of darkness before it rises and shines again. My women's groups have often had a good laugh about the fact that so many of their husbands have called them lunatics around P.M.S. time, without knowing the connection between women and the moon! So, once women have an understanding that it's O.K. to be as they are and to let feelings and emotion flow, I believe that **then and only then is it time to use the masculine principles of healing. These principles are imperative, but I believe so is the order of their use. They are the principles you would associate with using the power of your mind, your left brain. They give a definite and affirmative direction to the process of healing.**

Healing is about balancing these male and female principles within ourselves. Continued good health is about keeping them in balance. Then we can heal with **heart, passion, integrity and honesty.**

Summary of the Steps Towards Women's Healing

1. Acknowledgement.
2. Recognition that change is required.
3. Respectfully and gently releasing emotion.
4. Being honest with yourself.
5. Applying the skills of the mind–willpower.
6. Approaching healing with heart and passion.

Further Recommended Reading:

1. *You Can Fight For Your Life,* by Lawrence Le Shan, Ph.D. (Pub. by Jove, USA.)
2. *Love, Medicine and Miracles,* by Bernie Siegel, M.D. (Pub. by Harper Perennial.)

Now let us begin the healing journey!

What Change is Required?

Making the Transition from Silent Coper to Expressive Survivor

A woman's ability to communicate her feelings seems to be the result of two major influences. Her communication skills will depend upon her inherent nature and how much she has adapted and conditioned herself to her parents' behavioural patterns. These patterns then play a primary role in determining her actions, reactions and perceptions of life. Of course this greatly affects basic traits like communication and stress management skills.

In fact, for a woman, it is often the mother or prime female caregiver who will have the most influence on how these behavioural patterns develop.

It is quite probable that these same behavioural patterns can play a significant part in determining whether or not you may develop breast cancer. Dr. Caroline Thomas of Johns Hopkins Medical School has investigated this important subject, and found that high blood pressure, tuberculosis, heart attack, cancer and suicide are all illnesses that demonstrate clearly identifiable personality quirks twenty to thirty years or more *before* their onset. In other words our "life script," which is how at an early age we learn to behave in the world, may influence the type of illnesses that we have to deal with later in life.

If your mother had breast cancer, you may inherit a propensity to develop the disease, but this does not automatically mean that you will. Certain other factors must prevail in order for the disease to manifest itself. The "soil" must be ripe for the seed to germinate! Lifestyle and behavioural factors are implicated here. For example, unresolved or prolonged stress, sudden shocks, unresolved grief and poor nutrition are thought to be just a few of the factors involved in activating cancer inducing genes. It has also been recognised that these genes can correct themselves again given the right environment.

If you have grown up in a household where feelings were not demonstrated or expressed, and your mother's method of dealing with negative emotions was to suppress them to keep the peace, you may have inherited the same coping characteristics without even being aware of it.

There is no right or wrong in this situation and certainly no need for blame; for this is the cycle of human nature. However, rather than blame, we can choose to come to a point of understanding—our mothers used this behaviour to survive as best they could at the time. But, if we have this same pattern of suppressing emotions, are we still following a pattern of behaviour that is outdated and no longer appropriate in our current lifestyle? And if so, what can we do about it?

Some of us may have had mothers who, for unknown reasons, could not supply us with our emotional or soul needs. So we have grown up learning to become resilient and to silently bear the inner suffering of the unmothered child. I have known women in their sixties who have not mourned this feeling of separation until their soul has demanded it by manifesting physical symptoms or generalised emotional problems. There is a lot of grief in being an unmothered child. For some women dealing with breast cancer it has been a great relief to eventually talk of such things.

The following story highlights such an issue. The value of communication, of expressing these significant life events, of bringing them from the inside of one's self to the outside, seems to have a huge impact on people's general wellbeing. The importance of this in the healing of illness I believe to be very significant.

Dulcie's Story

Dulcie developed breast cancer at the age of 48. Her mother and sister, had both died from the disease at the age of 50.

During group discussions about these behavioural patterns, Dulcie had realised that both her sister and herself were women of silence. They were well trained to "not make waves," as Dulcie put it. Their dad had been an alcoholic who was easily angered and would become violent if provoked while in a drunken state. Mother's advice had always been to keep quiet and not tell anyone about what was happening at home. These sisters secretly held on to the silence and the shame and stored it in the place known as the "void." Dulcie recognised this place immediately when it was described to her and she indicated to the group where she felt it. She sadly placed her hand over her heart.

Dulcie lived on for 9 more years but ultimately she succumbed to the disease. I believe she had a peaceful and dignified death according to a friend who was with her. The friend told me a little while after that she believed that although Dulcie died, she died a healed woman with no unfinished business to attend to.

The Unmothered Child and The Need For Nurturing

Who nurtures the nurturers?

Mothering and nurturing from the outside world is essential to us all. You may remember that there were four wise women who contributed to the feeding of my heart and soul during difficult times in my life. These women definitely filled, although sometimes briefly, a motherly role which involved sharing wisdom and care.

If you have lacked the nurturing in your own early life it may be that you have matured with those early needs still unmet. Your reaction to this may be the same as many other women—the nurturing that you give out to others may overflow to excess. For you know the emotional pain of feeling the lack of love in your life. So, you give out, attempting to make it right, making sure everyone else's needs are taken care of—everyone's that is, except your own. Somehow your own emotions fade into the background. But the nurturer needs nurturing, your breast cancer is telling you that. It's time to pay attention to you.

I believe that nurturing is particularly essential if you are recovering from breast cancer. **Breast cancer could be described best as an illness characterised by the misdirection or damming up of nurturing energies within breast tissue.**

A woman can carry deep wounds that result from a lack of nurturing. There may be feelings of grief, abandonment and helplessness in her life. Often she cannot identify where the feelings or longings originated from, there is just a sense of being ill at ease, empty—the feeling of "the void."

If you tap into this and find an awareness or a memory of being an unmothered child, it may now be time to heal the wounds. Cold, difficult or unsatisfactory relationships with your mother can be healed. After you acknowledge that there is a problem, the next step is to begin to communicate. Again, this is where a story can be helpful. Asking your mother questions about her own story can be a wonderful way to gain insight into her life. Often listening to your mother's story, can stir compassion in your heart and understanding in your mind of what she has gone through in order to survive. Importantly for you, it can give you incredible insights into your own behaviour. It is possible to heal two individuals as well as a relationship by listening to one simple story.

If your mother is no longer alive but you feel the need to heal the relationship, this can be done by asking friends, neighbours or relatives about your mother. Gathering some old family snapshots can help jog memories as well as connecting you into your mother's life and maybe other women in your lineage.

Through the process of prayer and meditation you can then proceed to heal old wounds, let go of negative past influences and choose via understanding and compassion the way of forgiveness. This process can allow you to recognise how and why your life skills have developed in particular ways and what you can do about improving them. Prayer and meditation are good spiritual partners and provide us with our most important communication in life—the communication between us and the Great Mystery. Prayer is the direct request for help and guidance with earthly problems. Meditation is the time spent in waiting for the answer in sacred solitude. I believe that the ordeals that life presents do not have punishment as their goal, but transformation. So if you have gathered a sense of the injustice of life or have a victim consciousness, prayer and meditation can be a time to release these old patterns, forgive and move on. The issues of prayer, meditation and forgiveness will be further explored in a later chapter.

The Role of Women of Wisdom

If you are one of the strong, gentle and silent women with breast cancer seeking wise counsel, support and nurturing, the appearance of wise and understanding women in your life will be a blessing. These women can help you to revive your creative life, show you the way with a gentle and guiding hand and help you to reconnect with your inner self. They are women who are initiated into life and know how to keep the balance of the two worlds—the intellect and the intuition. You may be surprised where you can find them! Usually, they are of the world, initiated by the fires of life and forged into tempered steel; yet strangely they also have a softness.

Seek the company of such women on your healing journey, for they will help you to speak your truth. They are survivors themselves who can teach you how to creatively deal with major life issues. It may be that your natural mother is the one with whom you need to connect with, but more than likely it will be strangers who fill the role, even if your relationship with your mother is a happy and loving one.

For regular support I recommend also that you seek the company of a women's circle. Such circles are once again rising in popularity as women recognise the importance of sisterly bonding in their lives and understand their feminine nature and needs. Basically, women need women with whom they can communicate, trust, and share the experience of living a passionate life.

Also, it will be very helpful to find out where your nearest Cancer Support Group operates from and attend regularly. At such venues you are likely to meet other women going through similar experiences to yourself and also women—wise women—who have walked the path of cancer and survived.

Further Recommended Reading:

1. *You Can Conquer Cancer,* by Ian Gawler (Pub. by Hill of Content, Melbourne, Australia.)
2. *The Healing Path,* by Marc Ian Barasch (Pub. by Tarcher/ Putnam.)

Chapter Seven

The Healing Power of Story

The wisdom of the Storyteller is the art of remembering.

The wisdom of the story is the image or the symbol.

The result is the healing.

The most helpful initial intervention for a woman dealing with breast cancer is to provide her with the opportunity and the space to tell her own story. The externalising of one's life experience in story allows for a personal review. With this comes a reorientation of your position and place in life, as well as an acknowledgement of the past. Story is also a natural and gentle way of accessing memory in a non threatening way.

Take a moment to consider how your personal history, your story or past is affecting your current life. Your perceptions, actions and reactions to life are all coloured by your past. This will be so whether that past has been a basically happy one or a life of traumatic events that has stripped you of passion and enthusiasm.

One quality of survivors who tell their story is that they can speak of their experience, no matter how traumatic it was, with a focus on the lessons they learned in facing the major challenge in their life. They can speak with authority about their survival, look for the good in all experiences and talk of how they have come through with new abilities and strengths that had neither been used or recognised before.

Over the years we have had many survivors of P.O.W. camps from World War Two who have attended our programs. Their often courageous stories, humbly recounted and told with great feeling, have provided precious insights into the mechanisms of survival. One hero or survivor coming along and sharing their story can provide a wealth of useful information, but more important is the hope and inspiration that the power of their story can generate. The ability of survivors not to be victims, but to thrive in whatever circumstances with dignity and self assurance, show true qualities of soulforce in action.

Try to read as many inspiring stories of this nature that you can, for we all have the qualities of survivors within us just waiting to be awoken. When our inner life is paralysed by emotions such as fear and anxiety, the power of story can cut a path directly through, causing movement within. Especially if the story is well told, the imagination, where the magic of imagery dwells, becomes alive. The joy of story is that the process can bring about transformations in a non-threatening and non-judgemental manner. For the storyteller or writer remains impersonal, like silent teachers whose blackboard is the psyche and whose chalks are the vibrant colours of your soul. Such storytellers are creating the inner landscapes of image.

Story and image bring a sense of aliveness and inner connectedness to healing. Importantly for the woman with breast cancer, when those stories are real, they become like beacons of hope on the stormy sea of life.

The Function of Stories in Cancer Support Groups

Imagine a room filled with 20 people all 40 years of age; some of them born Italian, some Jewish, Indian, Australian and British. Think of their diverse backgrounds with different cultures, belief systems, religions, social interactions, dietary habits and so on. How could there be one approach or system that could deal with such a diverse range of past experience? In an effective support group, however, they would all have an opportunity to tell their story to listening ears so that an understanding would evolve of how they have come to be in their present life circumstances. Sometimes during the telling of these stories heads would nod as other people in the group catch glimpses of their own life journey passing before them.

There is relevance in acknowledging the past. It is like following a detailed map that shows you how you arrived at your destination. This information then provides you with a direction, an indication of how you might make the rest of the journey.

Some may require the assistance of a counsellor, but often the collective wisdom of the group will provide a safety net of wisdom to support and understand their pain and their story. If we take the example of the group above, just consider the collective amount of "wisdom years" in the room … 20 people x 40 years = 800 collective years of life experience and wisdom! It is the equivalent of an 800 year old counsellor! It is extraordinary how often this collective wisdom is sufficient, in that it helps to provide a safe space into which people can expand and tell their story as if they are the most important people in the world.

Often the storyteller is surprised by the key events in their lives being expressed so openly. Isolated events that on their own would be impressive to listen to are often only small segments of the whole story of someone's life. Sometimes the stories are recounted in detail; other times they are merely fleeting feelings and wispy memories of events too painful to remember in detail. However, once expression begins, these events are brought to conscious awareness and the process of healing can begin.

What stays in the deep, dark cavern of the psyche cannot have access to the light of healing, hence the importance of expression and communication in relevance to recovery.

A personal story at this point will provide an understanding of this from the patient's point of view.

Debbie's Story (Recorded in June 1990)

"Two years after a mastectomy I am feeling better than I have ever felt in my life. For the first time I am at peace. No moment in the day is taken for granted. I am happy to live my life. I am aware it is a gift. I attended a program at The Gawler Foundation in 1988, six months after my operation. It took the best part of two years to recover from the shock and at the time of the program I was still feeling fragile. I was not sure that I wanted to go into a situation where I would be surrounded by people who are ill. But the experience was quite the contrary. The feeling was positive and friendly.

People became very close and experienced friendship in a way that they had never known before. I shall never forget the warmth and love, the stories we shared and the inspiration, and the feeling of well being that this brought."

(**Footnote:** Debbie remains in good health)

Stories that Heal

The power of stories to heal has been recognised and practised by healers and Shamans of all cultures for thousands of years. Some cultures today still hold sacred their art of storytelling. For them it is a way of life. It is a way of passing on to younger generations, the tribal wisdom that has been gathered. Also in tribal cultures, myths and story are used to reinforce social behaviour and reinforce the belief systems that are an integral part of the structure and survival of the people.

Unfortunately, many modern cultures have dispensed stories into the realm of children's learning and entertainment. But have you ever noticed how adults really enjoy themselves when reading classic fairytales or adventure stories to children? There is a simplicity in these stories and yet their symbols and messages can be quite profound. We all tend to remember the stories that touched us deeply in childhood and when we read them to a child it is always fascinating to see how they bring memories flooding back.

In writing about this I am reminded of the biblical quote regarding healing.

"In order to heal ye must be as little children."

Stories can take us back to that state of uncluttered mind where healing images can simply communicate their messages. Some stories are archetypal in nature, with powerful messages carried in words, symbols and images. These stories reach to places within that otherwise would be inaccessible. Fairy tales, fables and parables are certainly in this realm.

This is why today many people are reviving the "story" within their cultural heritage. They are reconnecting with a power that enables survival and they are reinforcing their spiritual belief systems. The Women's Movement and the Men's Movement are both using the power of story to reconnect with the precious lineage of the feminine and the masculine.

Stories, by way of their ability to gain access into the inner psyche, can act as catalysts to initiate change. Images and symbols are the language of this realm and although healing requires the use of both masculine and feminine qualities, it seems that women often have a more immediate and direct connection with the use of story and imagery. This is probably due to the fact that women are seen to have a predominance of right brain function which is the intuitive and creative side of the brain. Men can find it difficult if they do not easily have access to creativity in their life, but it is a skill which can be learnt.

Life is an act of constantly balancing our feminine forces of creativity with the masculine forces of will. We all possess these male and female aspects and they are symbolised as the intuition and the intellect. Often there is a struggle and a resulting inner chaos if we get these principles out of balance for any long period of time.

For instance, a working mother who is a business executive may find that to survive in a male environment she must use will, decisiveness and aggression in order to be competitive with her peers. This can cause a woman all sorts of problems as her nurturing and intuitive side are forced into the background. I have seen this pattern in many younger women dealing with breast cancer. You can see that although their story is different to those of other women we have spoken of, the key issue still centres around misdirected nurturing. These women are often highly stressed and out of adrenaline. They are often suffering from complete exhaustion and fatigue. Usually they have been operating under immense pressure and their suffering is of an intense and silent nature. But, once diagnosed, having the pattern of being the "doers" and achievers in life, they are usually highly self-motivated and embrace creative healing techniques. Recovery for these women essentially requires time out to balance their outer life with their inner life. For these women too, the use of stories that relate to the recovery of the feminine can be very helpful.

A Tale of Transformational Healing

Suffering, healing, change and forgiveness are the lessons of the following Moroccan Tale which is one of my favourite "lesson" stories. By the way, do not be put off by the title!

> ***The Stoning***
>
> *Once upon a time, a husband left his wife and home to go on a pilgrimage, as was the custom of their people. Before he departed the man went to his brother, who was a judge, and asked him to look after his wife.*

"Gladly," said the brother. As soon as the husband left, the judge went to the wife. "This is my chance!" he thought, because he had long coveted his brother's wife. The judge brought a gift with him and knocked at the door. The wife was no fool; she knew what her brother-in-law wanted and turned him away.

Undaunted, the judge returned the next day with an even more costly gift. But the wife only scolded him. "What are you doing?" she exclaimed. "I am your brother's wife. Have you no shame?"

Angered by her words, the judge went to his court. Before the whole village he accused his sister-in-law of being a prostitute. The judge was an elegant speaker, and his words inflamed everyone. The people stormed the wife's house, dragged the innocent woman out, and threw stones at her until she collapsed. Then the villagers left her for dead.

A little later, a traveller passed by the pile of stones and heard moaning from within. He dug through the rocks and found the wife, barely breathing. The traveller took pity on her and carried her home to his own wife and family. The kind man and his wife nursed the injured woman back to health and invited her to stay with them.

When the wounded wife recovered, she found that she could heal the sick. She cured a neighbour's fever and gave sight back to a blind man. Word of her power spread throughout the land, and people came to her for their ailments. So the wife began a new life as a healer. Everyday she received the sick from behind a screen, hidden from view, and asked questions of her patients. Then she advised them on a cure, and all who came to her went away healed.

Meanwhile far away in his village, the judge succumbed to a grave illness. Ugly sores spread over his body and festered painfully. He summoned doctors and priests, but they could not cure him. The judge tried potions and lotions, and he prayed at all the holy places. But nothing worked. Day by day he grew weaker and more hideous.

The judge's brother finally returned from his pilgrimage. He found his house empty and hurried to his brother. "Where is my wife?" he exclaimed.

"She was stoned to death for being a prostitute!" the judge explained.

"What are you talking about?" the husband demanded. He could not believe his ears. But the judge and the villagers repeated the story.

"She is dead." the judge said. The husband was heartbroken, but there was nothing he could do. Then he noticed how ill his brother was. "On my travels," the husband said "I heard of a great healer who lives some distance from here. People say she can cure anybody. Let us go to her and see if she can heal you."

The judge agreed, and they set off together. When they arrived, the woman healer saw that the two men were her husband and his brother. But they did not recognise her because she sat behind her screen.

"Tell me about your illness," the wife asked, disguising her voice. The judge recounted his miseries and the remedies he had tried.

"The cause of this malady," the wife declared, "is a grave sin you have committed. Confess this crime, or you cannot recover."

The sick man said, "I am a judge! I have committed no wrong!" The wife repeated, "Confess your sin, or you cannot be healed."

"I am innocent," the judge insisted.

The husband spoke up. "Brother, whatever it is, confess! Otherwise you will die from your horrible illness!"

Finally the judged stirred. Weeping with shame and remorse, he told his brother, "I coveted your wife, and when she rebuffed me, I accused her falsely of being a prostitute. So the villagers stoned her to death."

With those words, the wife drew aside the screen and stepped forward. The husband was amazed to see her. Then he ran to embrace her. The wife said, "I will cure your brother if you desire it."

The husband thought a moment and nodded. "My brother has suffered enough, and he has repented. Cure him if you can."

The wife went to the judge and healed him. His sores vanished, and he stood up from his stretcher. The wife and husband returned home in great happiness, while the judge followed behind—chastened and changed.

Stories such as "The Stoning" can give us profound insights into the nature of illness, recovery and transformation. Stories of this nature have been handed down over centuries and symbolize the reality of traumatic life encounters as well as providing the remedy, the healing and the lesson.

The wife in the story has been treated unfairly, firstly by being wrongly accused and then by being stoned. This symbolizes the "wounding," which no doubt is added to by the betrayal of the villagers. She is buried under a pile of stones and left for dead. She then dies the symbolic death (classically talked about in healing circles as the Shaman's death—a time when the old way of life ceases and a totally new way begins). She is found by a traveller and offered care and compassion. When she recovers, she has the power to heal the sick (transformation of the wounded healer). She then seeks to have her truth known and through transcendence and compassion, (the initiated wise woman) grants forgiveness and healing to the judge.

In relation to the journey of a woman with breast cancer, similar stages are passed through.

These are the Stages of the Emotional Healing of Breast Cancer

1. **Emotional "wounding"**
2. **Emotional and physical suffering**
3. **Symbolic death**
4. **Transformational healing**
5. **Initiation into the "wounded" healer**
6. **Wise woman: Giving healing, compassion and forgiveness, leading to revitalisation and renewal for all.**

I see these principles so often in my work. One woman who heals her breast cancer, having travelled through the dark tunnel of uncertainty herself, heals her life, heals her "wound" and becomes the one who can point the way for others.

Selecting Stories

When selecting stories for healing allow your intuition to guide you. You will know instantly when a story is relevant for you. It will touch a place deep within. You will be aware of a movement, a resonance within your being that brings an immediate recognition. In that moment you will know what needs paying attention to.

Sometimes stories appropriate to your need or your illness will be replicated, or appear symbolically during your sleeping dreams. Be grateful for them if they do for they will surely have significance for you.

Remember too, that stories are not given to us by The Storyteller from the village any more, but are more likely to be presented to us in ready made images such as in film and television. According to some American studies that were conducted a few years ago, the powerful images of film can effect the functioning and status of our immune system.

Immunological tests were conducted before and after viewing of the films and followed up for a period of one month. Two films were used in the study, one a light and happy film and the other a horror film. Researchers found that the effects of the happy movie gave significant increases in immune function. However, the horror movie group saw corresponding, significant negative decreases in their immunity.

You may be familiar with the story of Norman Cousins, who many years ago was diagnosed with ankylosing spondylitis, a crippling and painful bone disease. Norman recognised the power of humour and image in healing, so he had Marx Brothers and Charlie Chaplin movies brought into the hospital to help him manage. He was also one of the first people to be very public about the use of intravenous vitamin C in his healing. Norman laughed his way out of pain and back to health. His books make inspiring reading for anyone dealing with illness.

I would suggest that "feel good" movies are a wise choice. Use the power of story to every advantage, and with literature, choose positive reading that will inspire and amuse rather than depress you.

In conclusion I will leave you with an old Hasidic proverb that tells us something of the power of story to heal.

> *Give people a fact or an idea; and you enlighten their minds;*
>
> *Give people a story and you touch their souls!*

Further recommended reading:

1. *Women Who Run with the Wolves,* by Clarissa Pinkola Estés (Pub. by Rider.)
2. *Once Upon a Midlife,* by Alan B. Chinen, M.D. (Pub. by Tarcher, USA.)
3. *Anatomy of an Illness,* by Norman Cousins (Pub. by Bantam.)

Chapter Eight

Using Your Head—Dealing With Stress And Its Effects

Stress would appear to be a part of day-to-day modern living. As we know, stress can be creatively beneficial or destructively negative. In order to deal with the negative stresses in our lives, it is not suggested that we attempt to live in a vacuum. We cannot eradicate stress nor can we practise meditation and simply make those negative stresses go away. Rather we need to develop a new view of stress and its role in our lives. Basically it comes back to a choice of how we wish to deal with the events in our life. On the one hand we could choose the path of viewing stress as a threat to our existence. This, however, is not a good choice given that we cannot eradicate stress from our lives. On the other hand, what we can do is to learn to view stress as a *manageable challenge or learning opportunity.*

Of course our logical mind can make a decision on this matter, however, when stress becomes a part of our day to day existence and we react to it, we become emotionally hooked. This is the pattern commonly known as the flight or fight response, originally a mechanism of life preservation. This instinctual response heightens senses allowing for rapid movement and sometimes incredible feats of strength on the spur of the moment. For example, this innate response will cause you to move rapidly out of the way of an oncoming bus. This response has a biochemical effect in the body, causing symptoms of pounding heartbeat, sweaty palms, shallow and rapid breathing, elevated blood pressure and various hormonal responses. It is an adrenal response and with it immune inhibiting hormones such as cortisol and adrenaline are released into our bloodstream.

If we view our human brain as a small computer, the flight or fight response would be like a program that was incorporated on the hard disk. As humans have evolved, our stressors have changed substantially since our program was installed on hard disk. From being chased by a sabre toothed tiger who was trying to make a meal of us eons ago, we are now in a hostile environment of a different kind. It is called modern living! With it comes all kinds of "mod cons" which, in theory, should be making our lives simpler, but instead the sabre toothed tiger is replaced by the debts we owe, unwelcome responsibilities and dysfunctional marriages, while our battles are fought on the freeways at the end of a stressful day.

Having acknowledged our situation, our story and our emotions, we probably will feel ready, in fact keen, to begin the process of actively rebuilding our health and planning for our future. There are many issues to consider.

Most of us unconsciously react to stress in our lives. In fact a good deal of it happens in the mind as a result of yesterday, last month or last year. There comes an expectation that tomorrow will be the same, nothing changes and so on it goes. But the brain can install software that is programmed with stress in the memory. That software is installed in the body. How much stress programming and for how long can the body run this program before the system breaks down or the wires short-circuit. This is why meditating in the body, reprogramming the muscle memory as in the exercise of progressive muscle relaxation is so important in the process of healing. To use the same analogy we can reformat and reprogram the software.

The opposite of the flight or fight response is what has become known as *The Relaxation Response*. This is best qualified as a state of being neutral, where balance and harmony are restored. It is the outbreath or sigh after the flight or fight response. It is the effect of letting go, as you will experience in the deep and profound state of meditation. Hence its importance in your healing program.

Stress and Immunity

As early as 1975, a group of researchers were gathering results of the effect of grief and bereavement on the immune system. They found that shock, the emotional pain of loss and a lack of the ability to cope with the profound life changes that sudden bereavement brings, all contribute to a significant drop in immune function. The part of the immune system which attacks foreign invaders and cancer cells, known as T cells, were seen to be significantly lower in bereaved people two months after the bereavement. Some patients in this study took up to fourteen months to recover full immune function again. Importantly this study was done with patients who were offered services of bereavement counselling. What is it like for people who have no support at all?

Since that study there have been many that have shown significant results regarding the impact of prolonged stress on the human body. In fact I read through some 2000 summaries of individual studies carried out in the area of mind–body medicine in deciding what to include in the appendix of this book. Today there is a staggeringly high number of published scientific papers in this area. Many journals are specifically focused on mind–body medicine, or pyschoneuroimmunology, as it's known in the world of medicine. The connection between the psyche, the nerves and the immune system, is no longer a wispy thought based on anecdotal information.

The Mind–Body Connection

How mind–body communication actually occurs has been the subject of intensive research since the early 1970's. We do know now how many aspects of this mechanism act. It is like a superhighway of communication, a network link that takes messages between brain, thought, emotions and body. This is made possible by tiny chemical brain components called neuropeptides. There are some 50–60 neuropeptides that have so far been identified and their function is to lock on to receptors on the cells that potentiate or activate the immune response.

Basically this new understanding tells us that the brain "talks" to the immune system and the immune system "talks" to the brain. For example our bone marrow, thymus gland, and spleen are all laced with a network of nerve endings which contain receptors for these neurohormones, neurotransmitters, and other communication assistants like the neuropeptides. Our current knowledge of this communication process tells us that our immune system receives its commands from the brain. Importantly too, it tells us that our immune system can therefore be trained either to defend more vigilantly, or to "turn a blind eye," thereby paralysing the body's defence system.

Can you now begin to understand how the principles of positive thinking, attitudinal healing and meditation might work as a part of the mind–body connection? And, if we consider the case of breast cancer, which has a heavy hormonal imbalance as its cause, it seems that our state of mind, our coping skills, our thoughts, emotions and attitudes, have direct communication to oestrogens in our body. It seems it might not all be in the mind, however, it may well be that when you change your mind, you communicate with your body, and in so doing you can change your immune chemistry!

Immunity: Threat or Challenge?—The Choice is Ours

Women with breast cancer who respond to their illness as a life challenge, realising that their diagnosis faces them with their own mortality, will often be the women who begin to actively search for solutions outside of what orthodox medicine has to offer. These women find something to live for, quickly passing through the hopeless and helpless phase which may have been evident prior to diagnosis. Their cancer has given them an opportunity for profound change. Their immune systems respond accordingly for, as you will recall, the brain "talks" to the immune system and vice versa.

For women who remain hopeless and helpless with their spirit dulled, feeling constantly under threat, the path to recovery can be harder. With motivation lacking and maybe inadequate support systems or isolation, what kind of messages are being communicated between their brain and immune system? They are not likely to be life affirming ones!

Recommended Reading for Mind–Body Medicine and its Relationship to Healing

1. *The Healing Brain* by Robert Ornstein and David Sobel (pub. McMillan).

Fear: The Silent Killer

June, a patient in a recent group, told us how impressed she had been with the power of fear. One of June's friends, who was diagnosed with a cancer that was not as serious as her own, died the morning after the diagnosis. The friend apparently had responded with incredible fear to her situation!

In India there is a parable told that highlights the potency of fear in our lives. It is called:

The Devil and The Pilgim

One day the devil met a pilgrim walking along the roadside. The devil was rubbing his hands together, singing and very happy.

When the pilgrim asked him, "Devil, why are you so happy?" the devil replied: "Well, today I am going to kill ten thousand people."

"That's a tall order," said the pilgrim. "How could you possibly do that?"

"Oh, it is very easy if you know how," was the devil's reply. "All I have to do is kill one with cholera, and the rest will die of fear!"

Fear of illness and death are deeply woven into the fabric of our society. Fear provides extra fuel on which illness can flourish once it is diagnosed. As we have seen from the flight or fight response, fear can change body chemistry significantly, sending out the danger alarm in a way that can get out of control and accumulate. Eventually this can lead to an impaired response from our immune system to foreign invaders and cancer cells.

You may find it helpful to consider how you are responding to fear in your life. Recognise if this is an area you need help with. For women dealing with breast cancer, fear can be a paralysing emotion, so much so that the fear can become the disease. Meditation can help with diminishing fear in your life. The "observer" can bring fears to your attention and help find solutions. **Positive emotions such as love, should be prescribed in large quantities for women with breast cancer. Love has a wonderful capacity to dispel fear.**

The Positive Side of Fear

This statement may surprise you, however, fear initially can fill a positive role as a great motivator in our lives. It can move you into the will to survive mode, enabling you to consciously decide what to do about your diagnosis. Illness can provide an opportunity to change aspects of your life that you have put in the "too hard file." So many women have spoken to me of this, and of how their diagnosis came as a relief after a period of time where fear, dread and hopelessness had ruled their lives. Diagnosis for these women actually relieved their fear and gave them something concrete to focus on.

The story of Jan's courageous inner struggle to find healing may help you to understand these concepts on a practical level.

Jan's Story (May 1994)

"In July 1990 I had a mastectomy after a diagnosis of carcinoma of the breast. Five weeks later I returned to my work as a family therapist, working with children and families in violent and sexually abusive situations. This was a week after my husband had an emergency appendectomy. One month later he had a breakdown and would not return to full time work for six months. We were struggling in our 22 year old marriage. So I took up full time work and the following year took steps to start my Masters. I kept wondering if I had made enough changes to prevent getting secondaries, but I had made myself too busy to think too much about it.

"In May 1992, a 4cm x 8cm mass was discovered in the right lobe of my liver and 2cm ones were scattered throughout the left lobe. I felt utterly devastated and full of self blame for not making the necessary changes, full of guilt for the children's sakes and very angry. The doctors basically wrote me off, saying there was a very small chance that Tamoxifen would help, but I reluctantly decided to go on it. I re-read *"You Can Conquer Cancer"* by Ian Gawler and attended a Foundation program. I began to piece together an understanding of why I had got cancer in the first place and why I had got secondaries. There were so many factors including my perfectionist nature, living my life according to others' expectations, pleasing behaviours and feeling highly responsible that it was up to me to make people feel better and so on.

"It felt like months of misery combined with a sense of panic and I was concerned that I did not have the positive attitude I needed to heal myself. But, I was also aware for the first time, that **I was allowing myself to *feel* negative emotions** instead of burying and denying them as I had always done, *out of fear.*

"In January 1993, I decided to begin to face the prospect of death, moving past denial (oh it is so painful to face one's negativities) as a result of my terrible prognosis—30% live 2 years, 5% live 10 years. Sogyal Rimpoche's book, "The Tibetan Book of Living and Dying" helped me through this stage and I have no fear of death now.

"In April 1993, I attended another Gawler Foundation course, and once again I experienced more profound changes with the help of Foundation psychologist, Bob Sharples. He has been a wonderful support for me. I realised then that I could not return to part-time work and study as I had planned to. Whilst I felt well, I still needed to learn how to break the busy pattern of my life and be still and quiet. This was very traumatic as I faced my deep attachment to my identity as a therapist/senior team member/public servant. If I wasn't those things, who was I?

"Investigations in May 1993, showed that there were no tumours left in my liver! I was elated and had a party to thank all my friends and my poor parents who had been so distressed, for all their prayers and support. So many of their friends and relatives had prayed for my recovery.

"So, I gave it my all. Meditating for 3 hours per day, looking after my nutrition and having 5 or 6 juices per day, vitamin supplements, exercise, etc. 1993 was a very tough year as my daughter struggled with the separation and her fears about me dying, during her final year at school. I see now how much I tried to protect them and not let them know how distressed I was feeling so much of the time, and how guilty I felt for getting sick.

"I would do it differently now. Kids shouldn't be protected. They "know" anyway. It was a tough year too as I adjusted to living alone after 24 years, being a single parent, having no money, selling the family house and being like my former clients on a disability pension. I discovered I had no real sense of who I was after all the years of living according to others' expectations. In my healing I began to accept that obstacles are a part of life and they are a major opportunity for growth and transformation."

Accentuate the Positive to Eliminate the Negative

When cancer is the illness it becomes so easy to concentrate exclusively on its presence. So much so that patients can forget to appreciate how much of them is still functional.

During a group session recently, there was a woman whose entire lower abdominal organs had been removed. However, despite an incredible surgical history, she looked fantastic. There was still lots left of her that was well and functional. She told the group she had every intention of enjoying what was left! Considering what she had been through it would have been quite understandable for her to concentrate on her loss, but instead she chose to accent what she had left and enjoy life through new eyes: "a small price to pay," she said!

Breaking Out of the Mould

Most people with a garden will have old pot plants lying around that they always meant to plant out one day. If you do not own such a plant I would suggest that you go to your local nursery and buy a root bound plant. The nursery owner will no doubt be surprised! Ideally, have the plant in a terracotta pot. Take the plant out onto the path and give the pot one good thump on the concrete, cracking open the pot, exposing the twisted and inverted root system that tried to grow, but was not given the space to do so. Gently tease apart the roots noticing that even though they could not grow properly they have remained strong. Carefully and lovingly repot this plant, nurture and attend to it every day so that it now has the opportunity to live on.

Can you feel the relevance of the analogy to your own situation? Maybe your "roots" were bound and could not grow—but the "energy" of the growth had to go somewhere. Did it find its way to the breast, the area of our body used for nurturing, for feeding and sustenance of another being? Did the growth hormones oestrogen and progesterone get the wrong message and give signals to potentiate tissue to grow in the wrong place—like the bound roots that convoluted and grew back on themselves?

Remember cancer is not a foreign invader, it is the body's own cells that have grown out of control so they are not replicating to the body's blueprint. Cancer of the breast is breast tissue that makes primitively formed breast cells out of control—the wisdom of the body gone mad. Secondary growths of breast cancer show an even more crazy and disorganised pattern of existence by taking up residence in other body tissues producing primitive breast cells in bone, liver and lung tissue!

So once you have found an outlet for misdirected growth, the process of healing and reorganisation can begin. Be like the pot plant, break out of the mould, nurture yourself and heal.

Dealing With Negative Emotions as they Arise

Step one

When negative emotions arise within you, it can be helpful to immediately identify what the emotion is. If you have been practising meditation, you are likely to be able to find the areas in your body that are affected by stress. Your body can act like an emotional resonator, giving you the necessary feedback and indicating when your emotional state is having a physical response. Most people can relate to the feeling of "butterflies" in the stomach when they are nervous. The same principle operates for identifying areas of stress in the body.

Step two

Name the feeling or emotion. If resentment is the feeling, identify it by name and then ask yourself why you are experiencing it? Where are you feeling it in your body? Then ask yourself if the result of this resentment is worth hanging on to? Who will it damage? Recognise that you have a choice in how to deal with it. Do you consciously choose to hang on to the resentment or to let it go? This technique can give you an insight into your reactions. It may be that the feeling of resentment is totally justifiable. Many of the negative emotions can be justified, however the *secret* of dealing with them is to experience the emotion in the moment, and then not to hold on to it. **Let it go.**

Step three

Hanging on to negative emotions will literally "eat holes" in your body and cause those "knots in the soul" discussed earlier in the book. Just consider who will be the one to wear the damage—it will likely be you the resenter and not the resentee! When you consider it, the price of resentment is too high!

In situations like this, after your emotion is experienced and named, learn to use your breath, the outbreath, just as you learnt in the meditation technique.

Close your eyes, take a deep breath in and sigh out the breath, feeling the emotion in your body dissolve, dissipate. With each out breath consciously relax, allowing the breath to drop down into the body.

Now enter "the observer," who, without judgement, can discriminate the appropriate response. It can take control,

give wise counsel. It may say: How important is this to you really? LET IT GO!

We can then "drop off" the resentment rather than hang on and get "stuck" in it. This method works very well in all kinds of stressful situations and is like a method of short circuiting stress before it can take hold in the body.

But what if the resentment is old, or the people that caused the resentment are dead, and we still carry it with us? What then?

Forgiveness as a Solution—Letting Go of "Stuck" Emotional Patterns

Of course it sounds logical to the rational mind that forgiveness is a great idea. It really makes sense to let go of issues that we know will ultimately harm us. So why is forgiveness such a difficult thing for us to achieve? One reason commonly discussed in our groups is that by forgiving someone we may validate what they have done to us, making us a victim of their future actions. Others may think that revenge is justified and required, that there should be an eye for an eye and a tooth for a tooth!

It is a fact of human nature that revenge is sweeter than forgiveness. Think how many wars have been initiated by this one potent emotion. We are dealing here with a form of action that is inherent in our society, which is why it is so hard to deal with on a personal basis.

Another problem with forgiveness is that the negative emotions, like revenge and resentment, can give us a hold on people whom we *love* and whom we fear may abandon us. Resentment may allow us to hold on to relationship, even if the quality of that relationship is poor—to say the least. In some cases too it can be a case of better the devil you know than the one you do not!

It has been my experience that many women with breast cancer wrestle deeply with this problem. So many of these women who have been trying to cope, trying to be a perfect and loving wife, have had incredible issues to do with resentment and anger. Often these emotions have never been expressed. How long can they be held in the psyche before they are mirrored in the body?

Feeling betrayed is often another big issue. I see many women with breast cancer after the breakdown of a significant relationship which has led to either divorce or separation. Issues of prolonged stress, suspicion, shock, betrayal, loss of self esteem and resentment that are all withheld can blaze a trail towards illness.

The more I talk about forgiveness with groups of cancer patients, the more aware I become of so many different opinions of what forgiveness really is. Forgiveness is based on non-judgementalism and a premise that we are all essentially the same at the core of our being. The practice of forgiveness is a freeing process from which we can grow to a point of compassion and understanding. It can result in cutting the unpleasant ties that can bind us to others through the use of guilt and blame. Forgiveness involves us in setting boundaries in our life and defining what is acceptable for us. Forgiveness is ultimately an experience that will open up the pure loving energy of our heart.

When is Forgiveness Necessary?

In my experience, if an event or the results of an event are consciously dominating your life long after the incident is past, forgiveness, compassion, understanding and love are the remedies required.

Seek expert counselling if you are unconscious of what the issues are that are causing you to be ill at ease. All people being different and individual, means that some may need guidance and support along the way.

At first glance, all aspects of forgiveness sound good. The advantages appear to be loaded our way. So again, why is true forgiveness so difficult to practise? One of the biggest dilemmas for people who begin the practice of forgiveness is the realisation that when the forgiving is complete, the relationship with the person they have forgiven may change. With forgiveness comes a letting go. Once you have let go, both parties then have the freedom to choose either total acceptance or the freedom to move on in life—without carrying the excess baggage of guilt and blame with them.

If you have totally forgiven someone and they continue to repeat their mistakes again and again, you have in your original forgiveness set a precedent as to the type of behaviour that you are prepared to accept from this person. This is then your point of empowerment from which you choose your appropriate course of action. Forgiveness may result in a recognition that some of your relationships have not been life enhancing ones.

So, again, once you forgive someone you may have to let them go. To then trust that they will choose to maintain the relationship free of the bonds of resentment, guilt or shame—that is a trust which asks a lot of us! I think that this fear of lost relationship is why many people who think that they want to forgive, find it so hard in practise.

These are facts of life that do not seem to be acknowledged enough by many who write about forgiveness. Maybe working entirely with life threatening illness has given me a realistic view of how difficult it really is for these women to practise forgiveness. I feel it is so much easier to forgive when you are well, but so often we do not get the impetus or the inclination until we have physical symptoms to deal with. I have known patients to survive for several years hanging on to their resentments and denying their need for forgiveness. However, these are the same people who, on their deathbed, have seen the need to attend to this "unfinished business," let it go and heal their souls before moving into death.

So, to me it seems it is very much a personal choice as to the time we begin to forgive. But do be aware, it seems that to not attend to forgiveness in your life is like beginning a journey on a road that has a large boulder on it, blocking your way. The only way through is to shift it.

The practice of forgiveness is the way to the *heart* of the matter, the way to release your negative blocks to healing. It is an issue of personal choice, but one that goes beyond our mental processes. Where forgiveness is concerned, it is not what you mentally believe about it, but where and how you emotionally feel it, that makes the difference. When anger and resentment are held within us we become deaf to the language of our own heart. Accordingly, their release will give us an unmistakeable feeling, a sense of an opening of the heart and a warmth that could only be described as **pure love.**

J. Krishnamurti said of love:

> *"Of all the qualifications, Love is the most important, for if it strong enough in a man (or woman), it forces him (or her) to acquire all the rest, and all the rest without it would never be sufficient."*

Forgiveness will not eradicate the memories associated with negative events in your life. What it will do, however, is help to remove the emotional "sting" that often accompanies a negative memory. Like the removal of a bee-sting, it will be painful for a while, but then, as with the removal of a bee-sting, the inflammation and response will settle and the healing will begin.

Guilt and Shame

These two powerful negative emotions can keep women as silent prisoners, paralysed within their bodies. Issues associated with these emotions can reach way back into our lives and are very much involved with how we have felt, and feel now, about ourselves. Naturally they are also integrated with the practice of forgiveness, but this time it involves forgiveness of one's self.

When we carry guilt with us, we often deny it and our behaviour is the only key to identifying its presence. It makes itself known by the constant, unhealthy choices that we make in our lives. This will mirror in our day-to-day life as low self esteem. When this is the case we can easily be manipulated by others in our environment, which of course becomes a continuous life cycle. It is made more complex because guilt and shame, although unconsciously held within us, have the power to insidiously destroy us. Unhealthy guilt offers no promise of positive healing or transformation, but what it can do is to lead us further into other negative patterns of behaviour including depression.

It is my hope that the issues presented within the pages of this book can stimulate awareness of the importance of dealing with major life events in a positive way. It is quite a natural process when old emotions are woken up to have a sense of blame, guilt or some form of self punishment. Remember to be gentle with yourself, concentrating on the fact that you did your best at the time. It is important not to punish yourself even more. It may be that it is yourself who you will need to forgive first and foremost.

As children we may have carried the burden of guilt from our parents and voluntarily taken on the responsibility to heal the pain and to somehow try to make things right. Children often tend to do this to hide the real pain in their family life. It is a major issue for children of alcoholic parents to deal with. Often they had to put a lot of energy into trying to make it right at home, while at the same time trying to hide their shame and guilt from the outside world.

Guilt can only be dealt with and healed when it becomes accessible to the conscious mind. This awareness to the presence of guilt and shame can be difficult to work with initially due to the power of denial that accompanies it.

All of the negative emotions really need to be dealt with as a part of a healing program rather than as isolated events. You will find that on your individual healing path these issues may arise as a natural consequence of a process. For instance, it may be better for you if the issue of guilt were to come up during a meditation session, rather than being forcibly brought to your attention by a well-meaning therapist. Like images that come to us spontaneously, these issues that arise spontaneously are a part of the mind–body wisdom. When they arise naturally this wisdom is indicating that it is time for you to deal with the issue.

I have great faith in this system of spontaneous arising, because I believe that our inner wisdom will protect us so that we do not try to deal with too much too soon. By using meditation as your mainstay along with positive thinking, positive emotions and attitudinal healing, you will find that the process is gentler and your recovery more complete. Meditation practice in particular seems to provide the most positive and supportive backup for all the other healing processes.

For further reading on the practice of forgiveness I recommend the following books:

1. *Guilt Is The Teacher, Love Is The Lesson,* by Joan Borysenko (Pub. by Collins.)
2. *Say Goodbye To Guilt,* by Gerry Jampolsky (Pub. by Bantam.)
3. *Forgiveness—a Bold Choice for a Peaceful Heart,* by Robin Casarjian (pub. by Bantam.)

Chapter Nine

Meditation—The Inner Healer—Its Application To Breast Cancer

Meditation—Access to the Healer Within

I could not think of a better way to begin a chapter on meditation and its relevance to breast cancer than to give Julie, a survivor of the illness, an opportunity to share her story.

Julie was working as a nurse when breast cancer was diagnosed in 1983. Finding out about, and then practising the gentle art of meditation, had a profound effect on Julie's healing and life in general. She remains well to this day.

Julie's Story (Recorded June 1986)

"In September 1983 I had a mastectomy for breast cancer. The surgery was followed by a 5 week course of ray treatment. In August 1985 liver secondaries were identified in a routine liver scan and ultra sound. I was devastated—being a trained nurse, I fully understood the implications of the diagnosis. I was also angered that this should happen to me.

"My doctors felt that the cancer may be hormone sensitive and suggested an oopohorectomy (surgical removal of the ovaries) which was carried out a few days later. Soon afterwards I attended a meditation workshop with Ian Gawler. This was the best thing that I ever could have done for myself. I came away full of courage and thinking more positively than I had in years and I was determined to incorporate this into my life.

"I had read Ainslie Meares' *"Relief Without Drugs"* some years previously and had learned some relaxation techniques, but now I started meditating. After a few false starts, it didn't take me long to begin to have some success, although I had good days and bad days and only now feel able to slide into a state of meditation with relative ease. I meditated for about 2 hours per day—preceding the sessions with devotional reading and prayer. (Being a bit a of a backslider in the past, prayer was not always easy. I felt such a fraud daring to ask for help only when I was in trouble.)

"I visualised my body internally and turned my mind inwardly upon my cancer. I exhorted my body's defences to get cracking and reject this intruder. When driving alone in the car I talked non-stop to myself. I forbade my cancer to get any bigger, imagined it starving through lack of oestrogen.

"I awoke each morning with a realisation of dread, but **I had inner resources (God given) to overcome this and meditation to rely on. What a tool meditation is! It brought me to inner peace, comfort and courage. I was determined not to be too afraid of dying to enjoy the living.**

"Being a nurse was limiting to me—I didn't really believe a cure possible, but I believed and knew that with these new tools I now possessed I would live as long as possible with maximum quality.

"In November 1985, my doctor ordered another liver scan to see if the cancer was influenced by the oophorectomy and to check on its size.

"I couldn't believe it and no one else could, but there was no evidence of a progressive carcinoma, just some "scarring" on the site of the tumour. In April 1986 a further scan was done which was totally clear—even the scarring could not be detected.

"You can imagine how thankful I feel. My doctors are saying very little about the whole thing except that they feel it was the removal of my ovaries that did the trick! Up to a point, it must have helped, however, I know they are short-changing the value of meditation, positive thinking, etc. and I feel so frustrated at these attitudes. However, I will continue to uphold them in the hope that someone else can be helped.

"One doctor muttered that perhaps I never had secondaries. He was the same medico who had said of the original diagnosis that there couldn't possibly be a mistake (when I, in a state of denial, had queried it!)

"I will always continue to meditate and I wouldn't think of eating any other way. I have fully embraced the diet and controlled my sweet tooth.

"I feel so well and so fit. Life is better than ever. For the first time I've got my life together spiritually (belief in a higher being—in my case God), mentally (meditation and positive attitudes) and physically (diet, etc.) I feel just great."

Meditation: What Is It?

Meditation is a non-doing, non-striving activity that helps us to be focused in the experience of "now"—this present moment, this present time.

Meditation can mean many things to many different people. In attempting to define what the practice of meditation is, we need to look at the needs of the people using it. Commonly it is associated with spiritual pursuits in both Eastern and Western religious practices. But during the last twenty years, meditation seems to have taken a path into Western society, carrying with it benefits that can be realised and utilised in all aspects of physical, mental, emotional and spiritual health and even to enhance athletic performance. Other key aspects of meditation are that as a personal self-help technique it is readily available, you can take it with you anywhere, it has no harmful side effects, and it is free!

For our purposes, however, in dealing with breast cancer, we will concentrate on one type of meditation practice. For the purposes of restoring health, accelerating healing and stimulation of immunity. Importantly, we will also learn to use the techniques within the context of our daily life. Stress can then be managed utilising a natural process of meditation that will strengthen us on the inside and allow us on the outside **to wash away the negative stresses in our life—"like water off a duck's back." This is how we change the pattern of withholding to the pattern of letting go. Letting go of stress.**

So, our definition and method of meditation will be a practice that concentrates on the profound relaxation of the body and which, over a period of time, will lead to a stillness of the mind. Our tool to do this will be the progressive muscle relaxation exercise (P.M.R.).

Our aim will be to thoroughly concentrate on the body, after all that is where the stress patterns that we have experienced throughout our lives are held. Also, the body is where the illness is housed. Therefore, initially it is in the body that the deep relaxation needs to be experienced. It is in the body that we need to meditate. The experience of such a profound level of relaxation very quickly leads to a direct feeling of wellbeing.

Essentially the desire to meditate needs to come from you. It requires *motivation* and impulsion from the will initially, particularly if your feeling is one of being "stuck," powerless or helpless. To begin the practices of meditation, and to maintain your practice so that you feel its benefits, you will probably require *effort, perseverance* and *determination.* These may not be qualities that you would usually associate with the actual practice of the gentle art of meditation, however, they are **essential** as initiators to the process. Once this priority has been established, the results are attained through a method which actually involves a state of non-trying, non-striving and **letting go.**

When approached with an understanding and belief in its gentle power, meditation can assume its place at the top of your priorities list. I know of no other therapy that can so potently and positively affect every level of your being—

body, mind, emotions, and spirit. More than a technique, or therapy however, meditation soon becomes a way of life.

Meditation can also be there to help us to die well, when our time comes—how ever many years away that may be. A peaceful death with ease and dignity has been the experience of so many who have chosen meditation as their way of life.

Often those new to meditation can experience a sense of frustration at not being able to still the mind immediately. However, a method of meditation that begins its work in the body first, can have effects that are quickly noticed. In particular, women often will notice immediate help with relief from fatigue and insomnia. Noticeable benefits early in your practice can encourage you to keep on. Those immediate benefits alone make meditation a worthwhile practice, however its benefits are much more, as you will learn in the following pages.

How to Begin a Practice of Meditation

Ideally choose a time of day, when having some time to yourself will be possible. Choose a place where distractions such as telephones, including mobile phones are out of range. Be creative and use an answerphone if necessary to get some quiet time. Many people, when they first begin meditation, find that using a walkman with comfortable earphones will help them to screen out background noise. You can use meditation tapes during the learning phase or you may like to use some relaxing classical music.

Once your meditation is established, however, you will no doubt find that noises come and go and do not bother you at all. Tapes can still be used occasionally, especially at times of heightened stress in your life when your concentration may be a little lacking. Of course, these stressful times are the times when your meditation needs to be a priority—the times when you need to practise the most.

Establishing a time of day that you can practise will give a rhythm and consistency to your meditation. While you are learning, it is best not to meditate at times close to appointments, school runs, etc., as when you are new to the practice, you may be concerned about going to sleep and become anxious about being on time. Meditation is an in-the-moment, present-time experience, which you will quickly learn to enjoy.

If you are normally a very active type of person, beginning with some exercise may be useful. You may find that a brisk walk around the block, in a park or maybe on a nearby beach will help you to meditate more effectively This can enable your muscles to let go, and relax more easily. "Walking out" some of the tension from your body just prior to your meditation session is the solution for active people whose muscles can tend to twitch and jump about during a relaxation period.

As you take up your position to commence your meditation, remind yourself of its purpose. You might make a simple affirmation like, "This is my time to relax, let go and allow healing to flow." Having done that, having set the attitude or atmosphere in which the meditation will take place, abandon any sense of striving or trying. This process is an effortless one.

To help with this process, find yourself a chair with a back and preferably arms, a chair that is not so comfortable that you nod off to sleep instead of meditating. Meditation is quite a conscious process carried out with awareness, whereas sleep is a process of being unconscious, unaware. You will definitely know the difference between sleep and meditative practice, as the former will cause you to feel tired and heavy when you have finished your session. The latter will give you a different quality of feeling, often a lightness, sometimes quite a sense of a heightened state of consciousness. You will feel enlivened, with a sense that time has passed by quite quickly.

However, do not be too suprised if you do go to sleep at the first few attempts at meditation. As fatigue, stress and busy-ness have been your reality, you may find that your body so welcomes the opportunity to consciously relax, that you will go into a deep and restful sleep. Go with the flow. For a week or so, you may need the rest and if concerned about it, set an alarm clock (with a gentle alarm) to conclude your session.

If you have a need, due to your physical state, to practise your meditation lying down on the floor or on a bed, by all means do so. Do be aware that the possibility of going to sleep is real. The technique of progressive muscle relaxation can be very helpful in dealing with pain and as well is a good way of "relaxing down" the body before bed. Be aware however, that the benefits of meditation and sleep are quite different.

Practising your meditation in the morning, rather than at the end of a busy day can be helpful. Meditation in the morning is like "charging your inner batteries" before the day begins. Meditation when you are tired, is more like catching up. It becomes more like maintenance work.

Using Your Time Effectively

It has been my experience with meditation practice that results can vary depending on the amount of time that you dedicate to it. The ranges seem to vary from 15–20 minutes per day for healthy people, up to three one hour sessions per day for those dealing with life threatening illness. Again, all people being individual means that the length of time required to produce the desired benefit will vary. Usually though, once you have "touched" the experience of such a profound state of rest, you are keen to keep going because it makes you feel so good.

My general recommendation for women with breast cancer is 3 x half hour sessions of meditation daily as a starting point, increasing the length of time as you feel the need and the benefit. This can also depend on the severity of the illness and the impact of medical treatments on your general health. We recommend strongly that meditation be practised throughout all your treatments and tests. It is well recognised that meditation, either on its own, or combined with imagery, can lead to the lessening of side effects quite dramatically. (See Appendix III for studies.)

Learning the Practice and Experiencing the Experience

Read and re-read this instructional section so that you can practise it fluently on your own. Take your time. You may like to use a favourite gentle classical piece of music—for example, Pachabel's Canon. Put on your earphones if necessary, and take up your position for meditation. You may also like to have someone close to you read the meditation for you, with your music playing softly in the background.

Each time you begin, just when you close your eyes affirm that: "This is my time for healing, may peace dwell in my heart."

1. ***Choose your place, a place where you can experience a sense of personal space.***
2. ***Sit in a chair, preferably one that has a solid back and a place to rest your neck. Otherwise sit your chair back against the wall and use a cushion behind your neck and head. It can also be helpful if the chair has arms upon which your own arms can rest.***
3. ***Place your feet flat upon the floor, about 12 inches (30cm) apart, hands and arms either gently resting on the arms of the chair, or easily placed in your lap. Feel your back against the back of the chair, your head resting on the back of the chair in a comfortable position. Your position should be symmetrical, and have a sense of presence. After all, you are taking time now to honour yourself! An image of the position that I found has***

helped many people, is the well known statue carving of Rameses II from the Egyptian temple of Abu Simbel. Most people know this proud statue. If you do not, take the time to find a picture of it in your local library. The position of your meditation practice is important.

4. *Remove glasses and preferably contact lenses. Allow your eyes to gently close.*
5. *With your eyes closed, really get a sense of the feelings in your body. Notice parts that feel soft and parts that feel tense. Parts that are warm and parts that are cooler. Almost as if you are scanning through your body with your inner senses, observe the quality of how you feel right now.*
6. *Notice too the feel and the rhythm of your breath as it moves in and out through the nostrils. Take a deep breath in and sigh out the breath, feeling as if it was "dropping down" or "washing down" through the body.*
7. *Now, in your own time, pay attention to the feeling of your feet on the floor. Move them a little. Notice the textures—the feeling of your slippers, socks or the contact of your feet with the floor. With your concentration focused on your feet, contract the toes, feeling them curl underneath—stretching them with toes curling and pointing upwards too. Then, very slowly and gently, allow the toes to uncurl. It is as if you were watching and sensing the feel of the unfolding of a rose in slow motion. Notice the feeling of the letting go.*
8. *Repeat this exercise of contracting muscles, holding the contraction, feeling what that is like, and then feel what it is like when the muscles let go.*

   TRY IT NOW AS YOU READ THIS.

   Do it with the large muscle groups in the calves of the legs, the thighs and the buttocks (like the pelvic floor exercise). Have a sense of what it is like when muscles begin to let go, noticing how they become softer, looser—they may even feel like they are smoothing out. Allow it ... go with it.

9. *Allow the tummy to fall forward under its own weight. Begin to notice the effortlessness of it all.*
10. *Take a few deep breaths in, sighing out the out breath, feeling it wash down, down through the body like gentle waves at the beach coming to shore and soaking down, down, sifting, and washing through the sand—sifting and washing through the body. Allow the muscles down either side of your spine to let go a little, keeping just enough of their solidness to keep your spine erect—no more than is required.*
11. *Bring the shoulders up towards the ears as if you were shrugging them. Hold them there for a moment and then allow them to slowly drop down, gently, gently, under their own weight.*
12. *Allow that feeling of letting go to move down and through the arms, into the hands, and out through the fingertips, noticing the sensations in the hands—maybe some warmth or tingling.*
13. *Allow your head and neck to move from side to side—gently and slowly—and from front to back—allow the head and neck to come back to a comfortable, natural point of balance—sigh out the breath once more.*
14. *Focus your attention on your face now. Contracting the muscles at the point of the jaw and then letting them go—lips now gently parted as if you were about to say ahhhh! Move around the area of the nose, across the cheeks, around and through the eyes—feeling the relaxation quite deeply through the eyes—through to the temples, the forehead and every muscle in the scalp...letting go.*

15. *Feel it all through the body, more and more. Take in some more deep breaths—letting go of the out breath. Go with it, surrender to it.*
16. *HAVE A LONG SILENT GAP WITH NO SELF TALK. USE THE OUTBREATH IF YOU GET DISTRACTED. LEARN TO ENJOY JUST BEING.*
17. *When it is time to bring your meditation to a close, be gentle with yourself. Take your time. Still keeping your eyes gently closed, begin to breathe more deeply—allow the hands and arms, legs and feet to stretch out. Importantly notice the quality of the feeling in your body. Give thanks for this time—and slowly open your eyes.*

I have made tapes for this type of meditation which combine flute, harp, sounds of running water and synthesizer. These are available from The Gawler Foundation should you desire to use them.

May meditation become a part of your life, to help you live well, enjoy the deliciousness of your own being and enhance your connectedness to the feminine principal and to the divine.

What to Expect from the Practice of Meditation

For our purposes, to practise meditation is to experience a profound relaxation, a stilling and quietening within the body.

One definite advantage of this method of meditation is that each session you have will be a cumulative experience, even though you may feel that you have not fully relaxed or you have had too many thoughts going around in your head.

The process of *learning to let go* will happen at every session, using the P.M.R. technique. Therefore over a period of time you will be gently changing the messages that have been going from the mind to the body. The message to the muscles now will be one of effortless ease. With this will come a feeling of peace and wellbeing.

Once we begin to establish this new pattern of response to stress, it is time to take it from the meditation room at home and "road-test" how it works for you out in the world. The benefits that you have established at home will stand you in good stead, but it is in your daily life that the meditation will go to work for you during and after your recovery.

If you choose to, you can go back to doing all the things you did before the diagnosis. The difference now will be that you will go back with a different attitude, and new ways of responding to the stresses in your life. And that is what will help to keep you well. If your pattern has been one of holding on, holding in, you can now operate with a different view—one of **letting go** in the face of stressful events and maintaining a personally satisfying state of **peace of mind.**

Noticing "The Observer"

In your meditation practice, you may have noticed there develops a sense of the observation of one's self. This is another key helper in taking meditation from the armchair into daily life. The end result of your meditation is a very practically orientated one! What would be meditation's real value if it did not have "stickability" and application to your life?

Being able to both observe your life and experience it at the same time brings with it great benefits. You will begin to notice how situations or people that used to bother you, or things you used to feel impelled to hold on to, no longer invoke a stress response. Because you have meditated **in the body** you will know the body very well, and the observer part of you will indicate if situations or people are getting at you. If this is the case, you will become aware of feeling the stress located somewhere in the body.

Often for women, the area of the solar plexus is where they will tend to feel these emotional "thumps." This area, you will remember from earlier chapters, is where women also feel "*the void.*" So, we find that meditative practice will lead us and support us through the transitions of emotional healing. It will help us to manage and to deal with some of the painful and difficult issues that will begin to appear out of the void, as we tread the path of living true to ourselves.

As the healing journey begins, we often discover the enormous amount of negative emotional baggage and the stony repressed silence that is housed within the void. Rather than put a "lid" on these emotions we may need to touch base with them, feel them for a moment and release them. **Let them go**—a process that many women have described to me as like taking a shower on the inside!

All sorts of emotional baggage may become apparent to our "observer." This "observer" quality may well see these emotional issues for what they are, recognising that they are not life enhancing for a woman who desires healing. There may be fear, anxiety, resentment, anger, rage, disappointment and so on that will now be able to be freed. You see, the antidotes for many of these emotions are the positive emotional qualities and feelings such as **love, forgiveness, faith, compassion, understanding and hope.** These positive qualities need to be able to reach into the very essence of our negative emotions in order to transform them.

With old emotions released and transformed, with day-to-day feelings and emotions experienced rather than held on to, women can really begin to reconnect with their innate and instinctual wisdom. This is a natural consequence when one begins to live true to one's self. With this comes the reawakening of a deep, inner feminine power. This power carries with it tremendous healing potential and opens the doorway into intuitive and inner knowing.

You may have begun to experience a sense of all this when you noticed the "observer," or heard the small, still voice within. This "observer" is never wrong. It is like a deep level of "gut feeling." Once you have recognised it and become reacquainted, you may remember that you knew it well as a child. As an adult, as you can build confidence in your relationship with it, it will become your inner wise counsel, your healer, your friend, your guardian angel.

This quality of the guardian angel is symbolised beautifully in the painting on the cover of this book.

Books I Recommend on the Subject of Meditation:

1. *Peace of Mind,* by Ian Gawler (pub. Hill of Content Melbourne.)
2. *The Relaxation Response,* by Herbert Benson M.D. (pub. Avon.)
3. *The Wealth Within,* by Ainslie Meares (pub. Hill of Content, Melbourne.)

Recommended Tapes:

The Gawler Foundation specialises in meditation tapes to help people affected by cancer. Please write for a brochure to **P. O. Box 77G, Yarra Junction, Victoria, Australia, 3797.**

Chapter Ten

Using the Will in Healing: Affirmations and Imagery

When we are ready to make plans and put them into action, we often need a mechanism to break with our old habits and establish new ones. This is where affirmations and imagery are so useful.

What are Affirmations?

All affirmations are commands. They are words of power. Affirmations are a simple, easily learnt means that you can use to move stagnant old belief systems and to stimulate new patterns of positive action. They are a great way to advance from feeling stuck to acting positively and effectively.

Affirmations have been a healing tool for thousands of years. Probably the oldest and most accessible place to find them in quantity is in the Bible, particularly in the sections related to healing.

An affirmation is usually a short sentence which summarises an important goal you have set yourself. To work best they need to be precise and usually they are repeated silently, out loud, or even better, sung with passion! The more you work with them, the more potent they become. Used effectively, affirmations can be invaluable for establishing new and more life-enhancing belief patterns.

How Do Affirmations Work?

Affirmations convert our good intentions into action! With the use of affirmations, our will, our good intention, has the means to act with force. When the will is directed through an affirmation with conviction and certainty, there is a high probability that the end result will be brought about.

Experience suggests that those affirmations that are made at a deep level of self, those made with utter certainty; those are the affirmations that bear fruit easily and will have spiritual merit. To make that type of affirmation requires clarity and confidence. These are qualities that are the natural product of quiet meditation. They can be helped by open communication, the telling of stories and wise counsel. Once you have the clarity and confidence, the affirmative will can go to work easily.

But what if you are not clear and confident yet? This is the time when using affirmations can be such a useful tool in your healing program, particularly if you are having difficulty changing an aspect of your life that you need or want to change.

In the chapter on how conditioning in early life affects our behaviour, we used the term premature cognitive commitment to explain how we encode certain behavioural patterns. Affirmations work by making a new pattern of "commitment," thereby establishing new belief systems to live by.

At first, it can take a great deal of will to apply and use affirmations, but once you become familiar with them, they can be a fun way of healing. A friend often talks about his own introduction to affirmations some 20 years ago. Continued ill health was really getting Lionel down and he was looking hard for answers when someone told him about the power of affirmations. Almost every part of his body was affected by various ailments, so he decided that he would sing to his body organs all through the day. He made up a little tune for the words that were, "My liver is lovely, my duodenum is delightful, my pancreas is perfect, my bowel is beautiful" and so on. This may sound cute and strange, however Lionel had 100% success in returning to full health and enjoyed himself in the process.

Another patient I knew many years ago was having a very difficult time dealing with an aggressive ulcerating carcinoma of the breast which had been unresponsive to treatment. Mavis was very enthusiastic about the use of affirmations and decided to empower the response of a herbal healing balm by using affirmations. In an almost ritual way she applied the balm gently onto the ulcerated area, affirming each time "Only good, healthy cells can live here—no one else is welcome!" During the day Mavis would gently place her hand over the area and repeat the same words. Combined with her enthusiastic approach to meditation in which she also affirmed her healing, Mavis managed to heal the ulcer within 3 weeks!

The process Mavis used to increase her healing response is known as **imprinting.** She had chosen her goal very clearly and then creatively worked towards it, establishing a belief in the area's ability to heal. The statement of intention was precise and direct, and Mavis was very clear about her goal. Importantly, that goal was stated in the present tense. These are all principles that are necessary to make affirmations work for you.

Simply stated, there are three basic principles for the effective use of affirmations. They must be:

1. In the present tense.
2. In the first person.
3. Target or goal orientated.

How to Make and Use Affirmations

There seems to be a flood of books on the market today suggesting affirmations to use. Ian's book *"Peace of Mind"* has a detailed section on the use of affirmations and imagery. While these can be helpful, my experience tells me that those affirmations that people design for themselves work best. You have a familiarity with the way you think, the symbols in life that are important to you, and your own storehouse of knowledge to draw upon. Therefore you may prefer to design your own affirmations utilising the three principles stated above.

Many of our patients ignite their creativity and compose wonderful, fun affirmations. Often we hear them being passionately sung from outside the shower blocks during our residential programs. The following one was composed by a group member. It runs to the tune of *"I am a fine musician."*

Now I am a positive person, I practise every day,
My cancer's disappearing, soon it will be gone away
Now, I am a positive person, I sing it in the shower,
For I am positively blooming, just like a little flower.

Now I am a positive person, I practise it with joy,
I look forward to my meal times and always say "oh boy!"
Now I am a positive person, I love this world we're in.
I love my fellow neighbour, myself and all my kin.

Suggestions for Creating and Writing Your Own Affirmations

1. Affirmations need to be stated in the first person, present tense, as if they are already achieved. So they need to begin with words like "I am" or "I have." They need to be in the "now."
2. The goal, the desired result of the affirmation, needs to be stated in a way that is brief, precise, accurate and complete.
3. Compose your affirmations with positive meaning. For example rather than using "I am not a negative person"

use the positive expression of "I am a positive person, now."

4. Give yourself an open ended time frame, i.e. don't pressure yourself to have a result by a certain time. You may achieve it quicker than you expect!
5. Use direct language—after all, affirmations are words of power or commands to yourself.
6. Use precise language, being specific in your outcome. A direct, focused and precise affirmation can make powerful shifts in your belief system.
7. Set realistic goals.The object is to assist you with the replacement or transformation of old belief systems into new belief systems. If your goals are too way out or unrealistic, your self doubt will immediately discard them. Base your goals on the best possible result that you can imagine and believe in.

Dealing With Negative "Self Talk"

Hopefully during the healing process you will begin to be aware of the messages, the "SELF TALK" messages that play in your head throughout the day. Often they sound as if you were listening to an internal, repetitive tape recorder. These messages that we give ourselves in the privacy of our own head, 24 hours per day, can make a difference to the effectiveness of our affirmations and imagery.

If you meditate for one hour each day where you use your affirmations and imagery, but demonstrate worry and fear fuelled by negative "self talk" for the other 23 hours, you cannot expect a wonderful result! These tools of healing cannot be used as you would use a drug—i.e. take one dose and forget about it. The process of healing requires observation and awareness of ourselves and our thought patterns throughout the day.

Negative self talk such as "You're not good enough," "You always do that the wrong way," "You can't heal," etc., may plague your thoughts at first. You will need to catch yourself before you fall, replacing the negative affirmations with positive ones. For example, "I always do things the right way now." and "I am worthy of healing now."

Initially you may find it difficult working with affirmations in that you will be making a statement in the present tense about an event or goal that has not happened yet. This, at first, may seem paradoxical or confusing. But if we begin to understand the ways in which our mind works, learns and relearns, affirmations do make sense and can be incorporated into our lives as powerful healing accessories.

You are not fooling yourself or being dishonest by affirming something that has not happened yet. The key issue is that deep within yourself, you have made a fundamental decision that it is time to change. You may not know how it will happen yet, but your **intention** to change is clear and definite. That intention, combined with words of power, will begin to make a change or a shift. In this process you are affirming the result you require. Once inner movement commences, the process of transformation begins to flow.

By using affirmations, we are **redirecting our attention**, choosing a new belief and expecting the changes to occur.

Imagery: Pictures From the Soul

Affirmations combine powerfully with the use of imagery. While affirmations involve the repetition of words, when we use imagery we repeat images in our mind. The techniques are well recognised by patients who have used them successfully and health workers who see their benefits regularly.

Orthodox Western medical science struggles to come to terms with the mechanisms that would explain how these processes work and their desire is to look for tangible reasons why. The observable fact for those who work in this field is that the techniques do, in fact, work. While aspects of their mechanism may remain mysterious, we certainly can understand a good deal about how they work.

If we look to history and the ancient healing practices of Shamanism, we will see that they have utilised the power of imagery in healing for thousands of years. All the great religions of the world have used combinations of imagery and prayer to strengthen or change belief systems and to bring about healing.

What is Imagery

Imagery is a two way mechanism through which we can communicate with the psyche. I believe it to be the link between spirit, mind and matter. From my own experience I have found that there are two distinctly different ways that we can use the power of imagery in our healing. We can use creative imagery or spontaneous imagery.

Creative Imagery

Firstly, we can induce or create an image in our mind by linking into thoughts of a past experience. Choosing to think about a happy past event will bring back memories in the form of pictures in our mind. We may associate other senses, such as sounds, fragrances or sensations with these memories.

You can get a clear idea of how this type of imagery works and how it affects the body by this simple experiment. In this thought-connected image you can keep your eyes open if you wish.

Simply think about a lemon—oval shaped, yellow in colour, freshly picked from the tree. Imagine holding the lemon and have a sense of its fragrance. Now, in your mind, take it into the kitchen and carefully cut it, allowing the bitter juice to flow out. Imagine then dipping your finger into the juice and tasting its tart flavour. By the end of this experiment, your salivary glands are probably well contracted and there will be excess saliva in your mouth. The words have created inner pictures that stirred a memory of a previous experience, and in doing so, produced a result in the body.

This experiment gives us direct experience of the mind–body connection and how it works as an interwoven, integrated system. It also leads to an understanding of the process that might be involved in how imagery, which is of the psyche or soul, can influence our immune system, which is of the body.

While choosing to create images like this can have many beneficial effects, to me it has a realm of fantasy about it. It is not my preferred type of imagery for use in healing.

What I do prefer, the second way, is to use those images that **spontaneously comes to us.**

Spontaneous Imagery

This is not a consciously induced process. There are images that can arise spontaneously at any time, but are more likely to appear during meditation, moments of quiet revery or during dreams. These are profound images direct from our psyche, our subconscious.

It seems likely that these images travel along a type of network which links our mind and body. Imagery is one of the key pathways that enables activation of this mind–body connection. Our memories, perceptions and emotions register as images in our mind and are then translated to the body. The body acts like a receptor; it accepts and responds to the messages received. When these messages are received over long periods of time, they can begin to change our body chemistry. Imagery then is like a coding process.

Because the mind–body connection is a two way communication system, spontaneous images can be generated in reverse. In other words, images can flow from the body to the mind. This communication can inform and report if there is something that needs to be brought to our attention. In the same way it can provide a solution to a problem. This solution can be in the form of a symbol which the mind can receive and interpret.

Imagery has many useful attributes for women dealing with breast cancer. It can help with physical healing on many levels—by directly dealing with the tumour itself, by accelerating recovery from surgery or alleviating the side effects of toxic treatments. Emotionally, imagery can help you very effectively to come to terms with fear and anxiety about treatment regimes. So, how do we do it?

There are three types of imagery that we can use.

Literal Imagery (A Type of Creative Imagery)

You can use images that you create in your mind, and direct by thought or will, to achieve the desired result. It seems that at least 75% of people can create this type of image when they choose to.

This first type of imagery is known as **literal imagery.** One very useful way of using this type of imagery is when you recreate situations in your mind as they might happen to you in real life—such as a trip to the dentist, or a visit to the doctor for injections that your may not find pleasant. In the safety of your own lounge room, or a therapist's room, you can then deal with any associated fears in your mind, far from the area where treatment would occur. Using imagery, you rehearse; you practise a favoured outcome.

For instance, many patients have found help from this technique in dealing with fears associated with chemotherapy or radiotherapy. This type of imagery is practised in a state of relaxation. Once you are feeling calm and relaxed, the scenes associated with your memories of chemotherapy are replayed in your mind. You run through the sequence of images until you reach the point where your feeling of being at ease, being comfortable, is lost. At that point a therapist will take the patient back to a place where calm is restored. During the next session steps are taken to go a little further, keeping within the patient's comfort zone. A skilled practitioner working with imagery in this way can improve a patient's quality of life dramatically, for often when fear is dissolved, many side effects lessen dramatically.

If you are dealing with breast cancer and you feel that this type of imagery could benefit you, seek the support of either a group working with imagery, or an individual practitioner for guidance on what will work best for you. This technique is also explained in detail in Ian's book *"Peace of Mind"*.

Another way to use Literal Imagery is at the end of each meditation session, you can create a positive image of yourself in good health. A photograph of a particularly happy time when you were radiant can be useful to reinforce this. I often recommend that women keep one, or several such photos at key places, so they can be savoured throughout the day. Such photographs will stimulate good memories and positive feelings.

When the process required in order to achieve your goal is clear, literal images are the best to use. Another woman who used this process was a pathologist named Maggie. Maggie attended a residential program last year keen to learn the art of imagery to deal with her myeloid leukaemia. Of course Maggie's occupation stood her in good stead to be able to literally image what was going on at a cellular level in her blood. She was able to imagine her cells with great precision and had a fun time with her healing, using as her mainstays, meditation and literal imagery.

However, most of us do not have the bio-chemical knowledge to carry out such imagery accurately enough, and with literal imagery, accuracy is vital. So, what do we do when we do not have a clear, literal image of what we want to happen?

Symbolic Imagery

To me this is the most interesting and extraordinary type of imagery. **Symbolic images may appear spontaneously or we may choose to create them.** Symbols are ideal when we have a clear intention of what we want to happen, but do not have a clear idea of how it happens. Because the literal process of healing is so complicated, very few people can use literal imagery accurately for healing. But they can use symbols to convey the conscious intention to the subconscious, in a way that it will be acted upon. Symbolic imagery can be a way of directing the subconscious healing processes into focused, effective action.

Symbols for the healing process can be consciously chosen, but they seem to be even more powerful when they arise spontaneously. Karen's story demonstrates the power of spontaneous symbolism.

Although Karen was having chemotherapy for her particularly aggressive breast cancer, the prognosis was poor. But, importantly for our example here, the fact that her images came to her spontaneously was a key factor. She told me that, as if on a video screen inside her head, during a meditation one day, there was a clear image of this huge bunch of grapes; nothing else! The image stayed for several minutes, until she finished her session. At our next consultation, she asked of the significance of this strange image, particularly as she did not even like grapes. She was finding the image quite distracting, but it would not go away. At this point Karen even questioned whether or not meditation was for her!

However, the significance of this image for her healing was immediately obvious to me and upon explanation, she became quite excited. The idea of symbolic imagery was quite new to her. She had tried to make fantasy pictures in her head before, but it seemed to only distract her from the relaxation she aimed for. Hence, feeling that imagery was not for her, she had given it up.

This image of a bunch of grapes clearly was symbolic of her breast cancer. At a cellular level, the grape skins were symbolic of the tough membranes around her tumour.

So, with a new view of how this imagery could help her, at each meditation session, and always in a profoundly relaxed state, Karen would visualise and peel each grape. By imagining peeling the grape skins away, Karen was assisting in the process of exposing the tumour to the action of the chemotherapy and her natural immunity. But the next frustration was that each time she went back, the grapes had grown a new skin which seemed tougher and harder to peel.

Look at the symbology here. The truly unique image that Karen's inner communication network had given her was awesome. As a practitioner, I could not have created such an effective and symbolic image for her.

I believe the process by which **spontaneous imagery** works, is that the body, in communication with the subconscious or deeper levels of our being, possibly at the soul level, "speaks" to us using the language of a symbol or picture.

In Karen's case it demonstrated how healing might take place in her body! Such is the body's innate wisdom. From a scientific point of view, it is well known that tumour density is one reason why chemotherapy has trouble gaining access to and penetrating a tumour's core. Tumours can also make chemicals which help to screen out chemotherapy over time. During this process the membrane or dense outer layer can become more impenetrable to the drugs that are used. In Karen's case, there was an amazing similarity between what was going on in her breast tumour in reality, and how the body–mind symbolised this to her.

To conclude Karen's story, she became enthusiastically creative and changed her imagery to only peeling one cluster of grapes at a time, paying attention to being really thorough. As well, in her mind, she nipped off small twigs from the grape clusters. As a result, the grapes began to rot, and in her mind she carried the debris to the weed heap and burned them.

The result was that Karen managed to shrink the tumour significantly. She was suddenly responding to her treatment, much to the surprise of her Oncologist. So improved was she, that the tumour was able to be debulked surgically, which had not been previously possible due to its extent.

Karen survived for some time, however the death of two other patients who had become close friends, distressed her greatly. Her health rapidly declined and her tumour recurred virulently soon after. She died within a matter of weeks after the death of her friends.

You may find that symbolic imagery will manifest spontaneously or as a result of contemplation. However, if you need to consciously choose an image, use ones that come to you naturally. It is my recommendation that you do not use someone else's images for your needs. It is likely that their body will be communicating what is right for them, not necessarily what is right for you.

With any type of imagery, if your have been using images geared at destroying the cancer, you also must pay attention to the eradication process of any debris that remains. Find a creative way to remove it from the body.

Finally, as a purely practical consideration, you need a way to make sure that the images you are using are accurate and complete. A good way to check out the entire process of your imagery is to draw it out on paper, including the mechanism of the "clean up team." If you are unsure of your images, consult a therapist working in this field. However, many women have told me that after drawing their image, it became obvious to them what was required. Husbands and families also often came up with helpful suggestions regarding how to put the image to work in the body.

Like all new skills, there can be some useful learning to do as well as experimenting for yourself, so seek some guidance with this form of healing from people who deal specifically with imagery and cancer. With meditation, you may find tapes helpful to induce a physically relaxed state, and in the stillness, either use your image consciously or allow a space for an image to come spontaneously.

Some Essential Helpful Hints for Symbolic Imagery are:

1. Imagine the cancer as weak, confused, disorganised and vulnerable.
2. Perceive your body's defences as being organised, powerful, purposeful and effective.
3. Images used should be vivid, clear and positive. Utilise all your senses in the process.
4. It is to your advantage to image your medical treatments as potent and effective against the cancer.
5. Remember to do the "clean up" process after your imagery.

Abstract Imagery

Abstract imagery involves the use of universal symbols. For healing, the images of flowing water and white light seem to be extremely helpful images to use. They are simple to understand and powerful in their mechanism. These images seem to have a wide appeal to women and can be tremendously helpful during treatment. Imagining chemotherapy being administered as an intravenous drip containing pure liquid white light that flows through the veins and arteries into the tumours, has been a very effective image for many women dealing with breast cancer.

Fresh flowing pure water also can work well. For instructions I recommend that a tape such as the one Ian has made is a good investment to get you started with both of these methods. Both water and light are very safe and pleasant images to use.

What To Do if Dark and Negative Images Appear

Like a bad dream or a nightmare, negative images can often be very potent and even sometimes a little scary. However, I have found them to be the exception more than the rule. Also, I do know that the message will almost always have some significance for you.

If disturbing negative images do occur, however, you must seek qualified guidance and I would recommend that a Jungian psychologist could be of great help here. I strongly suggest that you do not ignore persistent negative images. Sometimes the issues we have screened from consciousness, that appear shadowy and dark, can be the very ones that will lead us into the light.

How Do You Perceive Your Breast Cancer? —A Special Use for Imagery

How you personally view or perceive your breast cancer will have an influence on all your therapeutic approaches. A question that I ask of all my patients is, "how do you perceive your cancer, what does it mean to you, and how has it affected you?

The answer can help to give each person, as an individual, a directive as to where to start dealing with their breast cancer. The following is a list of women's different perceptions of what breast cancer represented or symbolised for them.

- A nuisance
- An opportunity for change
- A parasite
- An enemy
- A challenge
- Death
- Isolation and emptiness
- A part of them
- Punishment.

As you can see from the list above, the approaches for women who view their breast cancer so differently will need to cater for their individuality. These women could all have the same type of cancer, be treated with the same type of chemotherapy and yet, depending on **how they viewed their illness,** they could all respond differently.

The patient who viewed cancer as death has probably lost her spirit and her reason to be. The best that a therapist may be able to do is to help her die well. Contrast this with the patient who views her cancer as an opportunity to change. Such a woman is already displaying possibility thinking and is likely to do well with whatever modality of treatment she chooses.

It is important to realize that it is possible to change a negative image into a positive and more beneficial one. This can be done with outside help or by the patient's own determination. There are a lot of possibilities.

A good therapist can give you techniques and tools to help you along the way, but they cannot restore your will to live. Only **you** can make the decision to do that. **You can choose to heal with zeal. The only real freedom we have in life, is how we choose to respond to it.**

You can choose to respond actively and positively to breast cancer. By doing so you are virtually assured of improving your quality of life and there is good evidence that you increase your chances of survival significantly.

Further Recommended Reading:

1. *Peace of Mind,* by Ian Gawler (Pub. by Hill of Content, Melbourne, Australia.)
2. *Opening Your Inner "I"—Software for the Mind,* by Emmett E. Miller, M.D. (Pub. by Celestial Arts.)
3. *Getting Well Again,* by Carl O. Simoton, (Pub. by Bantam, N.Y.)

Chapter Eleven

The Menopause as a Path to Inner Wisdom

Menopause is usually a natural transition time in a woman's life, signifying major hormonal shifts. It can also be induced by cancer therapy treatments such as radiation therapy, chemotherapy and surgical removal of the ovaries. In the natural development of menopause there is a slow progression towards transition which may involve a period of up to a ten years of adaptation time as a woman moves into the next phase of her life. On the whole, it is quite possible for a woman to experience this change without too much drama. However, a woman's perception of what might be, her expectations, can cause significant worries.

In current Western society there are many unhelpful myths surrounding menopause. The medical system commonly approaches menopause as a pathological condition involving a shrivelling of the endocrine system. Contrast this with cultures like the Native American and Chinese which have no equivalent word for menopause in their language. In fact women in these cultures whose periods cease, became wise women or elders honoured for their life's knowledge. In our own culture, women with healthy bodies, minds and spirits can move into menopause with knowledge and understanding, progressing towards their time of mature wisdom.

However, there is no doubt that the scenario is quite different for women who experience an artificially created menopause. Invariably for them the changes are rapid and dramatic. The reasons for artificial menopause in today's society can be many. In early days of surgery, removal of ovaries and uterus was more common, as it was not realised that the organs of reproduction had extensive hormonal value in the body. Today it is known that there are 400 different cellular reactions of oestrogen alone in the integrated system of the body. Interference in these systems has wide-ranging effects.

Today it is known that some tumours of the breast can be given the impetus to grow by being stimulated by oestrogen, progesterone, androgen or prolactin, the hormone involved in breast development and lactation. A term commonly used for these types of tumours is that they are hormone-dependent. One medical response to this hormonal problem and its relation to breast cancer has been to shut down the hormonal production from the ovaries by their surgical removal or by chemical means. Occasionally, this is done via radiotherapy.

Surgical removal of the uterus is called a hysterectomy. A bi-lateral oophorectomy is the removal of two ovaries and a uni-lateral oophorectomy is the removal of one ovary. If you are recommended to have reproductive surgery such as this, or already have had it performed, be sure that you are clear exactly what type of procedure you have undergone. Preferably ask your surgeon or gynaecologist for a complete explanation on paper. For it often amazes me that many of my female cancer patients are totally unaware of the nature of surgical procedures that have been performed on them. There have been a variety of reasons such as they have failed to ask at all, failed to ask the right questions, did not have the procedure explained to them in language that they could understand, or were too shocked to take any information on board despite an adequate explanation.

I have found it quite incredible that women could have such a sketchy view of what had happened to such an important part of their body. Maybe this too is linked to the *Women of Silence*. Many of these women were highly intelligent, but had given their power away—this time to modern medicine! By comparison male patients who come to our programs, seem to know an incredible amount about what has happened to them, and usually it is written down. Almost invariably they have a lot of knowledge medically about their illness. The men with prostate cancer are often very well informed. I have wondered about this a great deal. Could it be that women feel overwhelmed, devalued or embarrassed in a patriarchal medical system. I really do not know the answer to this! But if you are in this situation, do go back to your doctor and find out everything about your surgery and your treatment. The latter can be quite important in view of side effects from treatments.

Instant Menopause

Surgical menopause creates a "shock" to the body due to the ovarian blood supply being suddenly severed. Having your uterus removed is enough of a shock, but when both ovaries and uterus are removed, the shock to the body is enormous. This surgery creates instant menopause, a process remember, that would normally have a ten year prelude. I have seen women as young as twenty five who, not only have had to deal with breast cancer, but also premature menopause.

Naturally this requires major readjustments in many areas of your life especially in sexuality issues. Self esteem can suffer enormously and many emotional difficulties can arise. Usually around the time of diagnosis and surgery there is so much happening that not a great deal of attention is given to problems that may arise at a later date. It takes a mature relationship and a courageous woman to deal with many of these problems. Treatments are often unkind in their side effects and hair loss and nausea can diminish a woman's self esteem even more. Many women have commented that the shock of this instant menopause made them feel very much out of time or synchronicity with life, relationships and themselves generally.

Menopause would normally be viewed as a key transition time in a woman's life. At this time, as with P.M.S. or other times of major hormonal shifts in the body, there will be an emotional response. Many women falsely believe a myth that the ovaries cease to function at all at menopause, rather than the fact that the 10 year transition period is by definition exactly what it is—a transition of hormonal change, not a cessation. Whether menopause is induced or natural, this process can be likened to a change in electrical current. If it occurs naturally and gradually, it gives a woman time to adjust to this new way of being and thinking. There may be for some women, symptoms indicating that this process of change is underway. These can manifest as hot flushes which are nothing more than surges in oestrogen levels—like a boost of energy. They are not to be feared. Renaming them "power surges" in a flow of alternating current may help you to view them in a new way. Night sweats and mood swings are possible and for women with their reproductive system intact, heavy bleeding at times can occur. All of these are symptoms. They are not an illness, just symptoms of changeover time.

The more "stressed out" and fatigued you are at the time surrounding menopause and the more you have lived your life for others, the more symptoms you are likely to experience. I recommend that women find for themselves, either a gynaecologist or a G.P. with a special interest in women's health—someone whom you can trust and consult if any symptoms of menopause seem excessive. It is worth finding out about such doctors long before the time when you may need their services. Ask around and get personal recommendations from your friends. If you are dealing with a serious illness such as breast cancer, your choice of appropriate doctor may be life saving.

Now for women whose menopausal time is on "fast forward," all of these normal transitional symptoms are manifested almost instantaneously, with no preparation or adjustment period. Again it surprises me how many women do not discuss these inconveniences in their body functions and their sexuality with their doctors. There can often be a point of view that leads some women to an acceptance of symptoms that would send most of us running for help on one hand and running away from our men folk on the other.

Why do women suffer in silence at a time when relationship, closeness, warmth and intimacy are more needed than ever before in their life? This can be a very tough time for the partners of these women. Women who have had a diagnosis of breast cancer, and maybe the loss of a breast which threatened their womanhood as well, may now have to deal with an instant and early menopause. All of this can strike a blow at the heart of even the toughest survivor personality. Women I know who have lost breasts, as well as their reproductive system, have had to work so courageously and so hard to retrieve their femininity.

In my work I deal with these problems all the time, and interestingly, these topics are guarded in conversation during consultations, virtually never mentioned in a mixed group, yet always launched into with relish and sometimes even a bawdiness in "women only" groups! Amidst the safety of the group environment, where sisterhood and sharing of their membership and initiation into the "Scar Clan" is openly felt, women can at last feel free to share and question with understanding ears and hearts.

Some women openly share the fact that they have never enjoyed their sexuality anyway and that now they have an excuse not to feel guilty in denying they husbands sexual demands. This comment often receives a nervous and understanding chuckle from other group members and usually someone pipes up with a comment like "Yeh, I don't have to pretend I've got a headache any more!" Many women in these groups comment how they feel that their sex life in marriage has been more out of duty despite the fact that they love their husbands and this has always been a conflict for them.

These women often relate how they grew up with parents who were quite reserved or strict regarding sexuality. However, the majority of women I see are in the 35 to 50 year old age bracket. They also grew up in the era of more permissive sexuality and feminism. Yet somehow the old patterning and conditioning of their sexuality in the home environment over-rules all the information. I wonder if the generations to follow will be different and how this even might change illness patterns in our society? I wonder if the more open approach to sexuality will have the power to change the incidence of female cancers? Or will the old patterns still strongly assert their power? Only time will tell.

For other women, the story can be rosier. Certainly for some, breast cancer can cause their relationships to become deeper and more intimate and honest than ever. Often these are the women who have experienced long term loving relationships with a genuine level of care from their partners. Often for them, however, they have grown apart without noticing. A diagnosis of cancer has been a strong wake-up call for both of them about the preciousness of good relationship. They quickly embrace what our program has to offer, need little motivation, get on with it and enjoy their new life as Pauline's story shows us. It is fair to say, however, that in people who I see regularly, these couples are more the exception than the rule.

Pauline's Story

"In October 1987, I had a mastectomy and no further treatment. In October 1989, I was diagnosed as having extensive secondaries in my spine, skull, ribs and right leg. After three weeks of radiotherapy I was put on Tamoxifen. In February 1990, my husband and I attended a Gawler Foundation program, where we had an intensive week of meditation, positive thinking, looking at diet and generally how to live well with a life threatening illness.

"We returned home and put it all into practice. We took up meditation, became vegetarians and my husband gave up his managerial position to work part-time as a consultant and hence spend more time with me. I had given up my job straight after the secondaries were diagnosed."

In June 1990, Pauline wrote in a letter to us:

"I saw the Onco yesterday. Apparently he's a world authority on prostate and testicular cancer, so here's hoping he knows as much about bones as balls! A normally emotionless, but articulate man (it seems to go with the job), he had a lot of trouble disguising his excitement (he even looked as though he was gearing up for a hug!) and was almost reduced to a jibber on seeing my scan.

"According to him the report underestimated the dramatic changes since last October. He even gave me most of the credit as he felt the treatment was insignificant compared with my inner strength, building up an incredibly strong immune system and my support, etc. I had just returned from holidaying on Lord Howe Island where I had been hill climbing. Not bad for someone who was told that bushwalking would be off my list of activities.

The dividends have paid off, as I went into remission for sixteen months. My last two bone scans in February and June 1992 showed a slight progression of the disease, so I have been placed on another hormone preparation called Farlutal. I continue to keep very well. I am mobile and have little pain. I walk my dog on the beach daily, do my own gardening, (I gave the housework away a long time ago!), meditate daily and go to hydrotherapy and swim nearly a kilometre twice per week. I am currently planning a trip to England. So there is life and indeed a life quality after secondaries.

(Recorded June 1992).

At the time of writing, Pauline remains well.

The Menopause Story

The Myth

It is important to have an understanding of the cultural myths that surround menopause. The perceptions you have of menopause can have a huge impact on the outcome for yourself and your partner. Remember hormonal activity is happening in the brain all the time, whether you have got ovaries or not, and your view of yourself as a menopausal woman can make a difference as to whether the myths will fit or not. Perceptions here, really count.

From our early teens we were often told or heard about this condition called the menopause. We heard the good news and the bad news about it. The good being that it was a time when you could dispense with the "inconvenience" (as it is seen in our society) of sanitary napkins, tampons, and "bad" days. But the negative side drove fear into the hearts of myself and my friends who, as teenagers, understood that menopause was about becoming old, shrivelled, hairy and unattractive to men! Maybe the men-o-'pause' bit meant a long……pause from men! The inference was that after that time you were no longer of use to men. What an outrageous thought! But, subconsciously you know that thought is still there in both men and women.

This myth is often highlighted by drug company advertisements showing middle aged couples gazing wistfully out on to dry, parched cracked earth with some sort of slogan for hormone therapy next to it! If we, as women, buy into this cultural myth, no matter how menopause has been induced, we will take part in a self-fulfilling prophecy. Rather, I believe that by gaining a real understanding of the process, on all levels of our being, the result can be different. Our attained maturity, whether it be by age or by becoming initiated members of the "Scar Clan," can demonstrate the strength and the power and the beauty of women's wisdom.

Menopause: Revealing a Thin Veil Between Two Worlds

You may remember or still be aware of the times that are commonly called premenstrual syndrome or P.M.S. At this time, which is variable in its length for women, you commonly feel emotionally sensitive, maybe even teary. Comments are often made such as, "Look out, its hormone time again, better duck for cover." Or your husband looks at you in amazement and says, "You must have your period or you are out of your mind!" You may have even been branded a "lunatic!" which, as we have seen already, is an accurate statement, given that the moon's lunar cycles are related to women's cycles!

I believe, as do many other female health care practitioners today, that heightened emotional activity and sensitivity are normal in women at times of hormonal shifts. Menopause is not the only time in our lives that we have changeover of hormones—it has been happening all your life if you are a woman. Many women have experienced hot flushes, well before the time of menopause, because of major hormonal shifts. These shifts first happen around the time of puberty, when we get our periods, then premenstrually, during ovulation time, pregnancy, labour and delivery, breast feeding and of course, at menopause. The first 50 years or so is like sitting on a see saw of hormonal shifts and adjustments. The joy of being female!

Cultural perceptions and myths, along with a medical profession that is trained to believe that women have a reproductive system that needs fixing, are all factors that need to be looked at in the areas of women's health care.

There are two major aspects of our lives that seem to affect our hormonal patterns. These are the effects of prolonged and negative stress in our lives, and how true we are living our lives according to the tune of our own souls.

At all of these times of cyclic change, we as women become highly sensitive to any inconsistencies in our lives. Just for a moment imagine how that reframed thought gives a new meaning to all those times of seeming emotional darkness before a period arrives, and all the other times of hormonal change in your life. After I had realised this pattern in my own life, I felt freed from the myth that inferred it was a curse to be born female. I began to enjoy and take an interest in what was happening in my body and my life in a new way.

I believe that what happens at these times of hormonal flux is an opportunity for women to take time out, be still and listen to the needs of the inner self. It is as if at these times the veil between our two worlds of existence suddenly becomes thinner. For a woman, the closer her soul life is to being expressed in her physical life, the healthier she will be.

Many women describe these times in their hormonal lives as times when the intellect and intuition seem to face each other. It is highly likely that at this time, anything that is not right in your life will come closer to your attention, while at other times, these two worlds seem far apart and unrelated. Given the recent understandings of hormonal functions and the renaming of hormones as *messenger molecules,* I have begun to have a deeper understanding of how our hormones may act as messengers from our inner self, showing to us the inconsistencies in how we are living our lives.

These days I really make a point of listening to what my hormonal messages are telling me, rather than suppressing or ignoring them. I am also reminded of all the women with breast cancer, who have said to me that they felt their bodies were giving them *messages* long before the diagnosis of their cancer. To learn to utilise this aspect of what it is to be a woman, and listen to the wisdom of your inner self, is really what I believe to be your source of true power.

Treatments and Their Effects

Tamoxifen (Novladex or Novladex D) is a palliative treatment for breast cancer, an antioestrogen thought to work by binding oestrogen receptors at the cellular level. Trials with this preparation have not been extensive in premenopausal women as it is usually recommended in postmenopausal women, who have either reached natural menopause or have had surgical, chemical or radiation induced menopause. In premenopausal women with their ovaries intact, menstruation is suppressed if they are taking (Tamoxifen) for the treatment of breast cancers. But menopausal symptoms such as hot flushes, nausea and vomiting occur in about 25% of these women. Tamoxifen may be hazardous to a child's survival if a woman with breast cancer becomes pregnant. Vaginal discharges are quite common for women taking Tamoxifen, so regular gynaecological checks are recommended, especially when recent research has shown that some people who still have a uterus develop Tamoxifen-related endometrial cancer.

Tumours that have prolactin receptors tend to be hormone-dependent. They have a slower growth rate and are more likely to respond to Tamoxifen. According to recent information, it is thought that only 50% of oestrogen-dependent tumours respond to Tamoxifen. Two thirds of all breast tumours apparently do not respond to Tamoxifen, although these figures, as with many figures associated with cancer treatments, vary so much according to the research and the interpretation.

It can be quite confusing trying to sort through information on breast cancer. It seems to depend on which journal one reads as to what the answer might be. So in this broad range of information, you will notice that there are very few studies quoted through the text of this book. Rather I have given them an entire section of their own in Part Three—The Appendix, and have chosen for our purposes to draw on human life experiences for our inspiration, learning and emotional sustenance.

Chemotherapy

This type of treatment can have obvious short-term side effects, including hair loss, fatigue, nausea and/or vomiting, as well as reduced immune function, weight gain and menopausal symptoms. Some people even develop arthritis when chemotherapy is discontinued. As you can see from the lengthy list, natural functions as well as a woman's appearance and self esteem can really take a beating.

Again, I am suprised at how many women undergo aggressive treatment regimes without question, without second or third opinions or proper explanation of what to expect in the long term. Again there is often this silence, this passive acceptance.

But the problem certainly is complex. In London some years ago, a group of thirty doctors were given one woman's case study in order to suggest treatment regimes for her breast cancer. They came up with over 30 different treatment protocols for this one patient, all seen as valid treatments! So, basically it pays to shop around for the optimum treatment advice.

Drugs are commonly used in various combinations and they may also be used in conjunction with hormonal treatments like Tamoxifen. Ask for a detailed list of your treatment drugs and their possible side effects and take care to make wise decisions.

You may see yourself as a long-term survivor of cancer, but your doctor may not. It has often been said of my husband Ian, that statistically he should be dead. When the question of his survival has been spoken about, however, he is often described as an "anecdote." My answer to that is that I would rather be married to a live anecdote, than a dead statistic! Most secondary breast cancer treatments are still regarded as palliative, rather than curative treatments and quality of life and survival issues must be taken into account by you, the patient.

Dealing With Menopausal Symptoms

The combination for women with breast cancer of surfacing emotions, deep inner feelings and hormonal interplay can mean that there are a few symptoms to deal with. Unless menopausal symptoms are severe and interfering with your quality of life or maybe sleep patterns, they will tend to take care of themselves. Hot flushes, for instance, usually last for about six to nine months before the balance point is reached hormonally. For women experiencing normal menopause, it is thought that about 80% will experience what would be considered normal and manageable symptoms. These women are likely to find menopause a challenging experience that is bringing about changes in the way they think and act according to their inner wisdom. The other 20% are likely to be women who will need the help of a gynaecologist to deal with excessive symptoms. Adequate stress management techniques are also needed to assist these women in re establishing a normal balance to their lives.

Some of the problems seen to be associated with menopause are lowered oestrogen, linking with osteoporosis, some loss of protection for veins, arteries and heart, thinning of the vaginal walls leading to dryness, and sometimes painful inflammation, and as already mentioned, night sweats, hot flushes and mood swings.

Firstly, many women are unaware of the fact that their ovaries do not shut down completely at menopause. Ovaries provide women with hormones for the course of their entire life. Some studies have indicated that after menopause the ovaries actually produce more androgens than before. Our bodies are very clever—they have a wisdom. This wisdom allows an oestrogen, called oestrone, to be converted from cholesterol in a woman's body fat. Could it be nature's way of compensating women by supplying us at middle age with more body fat to help with hormonal output in the body when we are post menopausal?

Night sweats, sleeplessness and anxiety can be caused by lowered tryptophan levels that correspond with lowered oestrogen levels. Prescribed supplements, containing tryptophan taken a few hours before bedtime, can significantly reduce night sweats as well as helping with associated sleeplessness and anxiety.

Dryness of the vagina can also be caused by lowered oestrogen levels. These lower levels also tend to make the lining of the vagina thinner and therefore more easily damaged. This can be a problem, not only if you have a sex partner. The lining being dry and inflamed can be just plain uncomfortable. Some women are prescribed oestrogen creams, others use a lubricant like K.Y. Jelly as required, and others find a product named "Replens" useful. Replens is a non hormonal lubricant. Paying attention to good quality natural fats and oils in your diet is also helpful. Remember too, however, that all areas of the body that are not used will tend to atrophy and get smaller, the vagina is no exception. Using lubrication, with active participation in sex and a gentle partner can greatly improve the situation. You will need to have better communication about your sexual functioning with your partner than ever before. There are often solutions to even the most difficult of these problems. Ask your gynaecologist for a referral to see a specialist sex therapist or counsellor for help if you need it.

Hormone Replacement: Current Information

We need to keep in perspective that our current knowledge on women's hormonal cycles and menopause is still in embryonic stages. Women, prior to this century, spent most of their years pregnant and breast feeding, therefore they probably had very little menstrual activity or the experience of menopause at all. Many women died in their early forties in those days.

There is opposing evidence regarding the use of hormone replacement therapy in postmenopausal women. It is now known that ovarian hormones are provided for a woman for her entire life, that the ovaries do not cease to function, but rather change their function. As already mentioned it is now known that cholesterol can be converted from body fat into estrone, an oestrogen. In fact it is thought that 25% of the positive effects of oestrogen on the cardiovascular system are related to its ability to metabolise cholesterol in a woman's body.

It is now also known that these hormones not only have a localised effect in the body within the organs of reproduction, but are used systemically. It is now known that oestrogen is involved in 400 different cellular activities! The more that is discovered about these hormones or messenger molecules, the more we appreciate the body–mind as an incredibly integrated system. For example, due to its positive action on blood vessels, migraine can be relieved by the addition of oestrogen as it can release the constriction in blood flow.

As well as the protective effect on our heart, veins and arteries, oestrogens can also act in the body as free radical scavengers, or as they are commonly known, antioxidants. These substances protect our cells from damage and injury. Also well known is the positive effect of oestrogen on bone loss and halting osteoporosis, but this will be the subject of our next chapter.

When all of this is considered, it is not surprising that oestrogen deprivation may result in many functional irregularities within women. So it is easy to make a case for Hormone Replacement Therapy (HRT), especially in women who have had an induced early menopause. But still, it is open to conjecture, as some studies state a higher rate of breast cancer among women taking HRT, than those who do not. However, another remarkable and interesting thing was that women who did have breast cancer and who were on HRT, had a higher survival rate. It is also worth noting that women who have had an early menopause, have a statistically significant decreased risk of breast cancer. However, if you developed breast cancer premenopause, HRT may carry a risk due to the impact of excess oestrogen, so often it is not recommended. Your individual situation needs careful assessment and monitoring when dealing with HRT and breast cancer. This is another good reason to have a doctor with whom you can communicate well. The usual recommendation is to take the smallest amount that works and you may need professional advice to find an individual dose that works for you.

Oestrogen, when taken on its own (called unopposed oestrogen), caused a problem with cancer of the uterus in women many years ago. Of course this was only of concern to the women who still had their uterus intact. Progesterone was the missing ingredient which caused the lining of the uterus to build up, causing cancer. An artificial progestin is used today in conjunction with oestrogen.

It is a delicate matter of weighing up risks versus benefits with your doctor. If it does come to treatment, it is helpful for you to know that there are about twenty different combinations of HRT available. Armed with some information, you will be in a better position to discuss the possibilities with your doctor and work out your best course of action.

However, I cannot help but wonder about the wisdom we carry within us and how it might be better utilised. From my experience, women who adopt a regular practice of meditation and stress management do better taking the medical hormonal treatments than those who do not. Because of the positive, balancing effect that meditation can have on our brain chemistry and our hormones, which has been documented, I believe it is the one practice that can safely help women to achieve their own appropriate and individual hormonal balance, in conjunction with their medical treatment.

Suggestions For Managing Menopausal Symptoms

1. Lifestyle changes: Adopting a healthy lifestyle can have a huge impact on menopause management. A nutrient-dense diet is essential. Use a diet based on fruits, vegetables and grains. The emphasis should be on a high pro-

portion of fresh vegetables in your diet, especially the leafy greens. A diet that is high in fibre, low in fat, has a low to moderate protein intake and has a low intake of added salt, will increase your wellbeing substantially. Take care not to over load your system with excessive quantities of dairy food. Natural yoghurt, quark, leben and natural cheeses including cottage and ricotta cheeses, are healthy additions to the diet. Low fat content is preferable.

2. Remember, it is not only what you eat, but what your body does with what you eat. It has been found that many women over 40 show signs of low gastric acid secretion. This means that protein in particular, will not be able to be digested properly. There are plenty of natural products, rather than taking more tablets, that cater for this. For example, horseradish and ginger can be added as a part of your protein meal. I would suggest you ask your health therapist if this is important in your case.

   For a complete overview of nutrition and recommendations for cancer patients, see chapters 7 and 8 of *"You Can Conquer Cancer"* by Ian Gawler (Hill of Content, Melbourne, 1984.)

3. If you are having hot flushes, avoid all spicy foods, as they can make the symptoms more unpleasant.

4. Eliminate coffee, lower your alcohol intake to special occasions and deal with your smoking habit if you have one. Be sure not to stop smoking without replacing the habit with a more health-promoting one—a habit that will be life enhancing. This may mean that a new way of coping with stress in your life may be relevant, especially if you have used smoking as a stress management tool. Think carefully about what smoking means for you. An adequate healthy replacement habit could well be

just as important as giving up the smoking for health reasons.

5. Check with your doctor that other medications you are taking are not worsening any menopausal symptoms you may have. This can happen easily if you have attended more than one doctor and have not communicated other treatments you are having.
6. For complementary health care, do seek the advice of a professional in your chosen modality of treatment. Herbal medicines, homeopathics and other natural therapies will work best when prescribed for your individual needs and situation.
7. Tepid showers can be really helpful for instant management of hot flushes.
8. On a nutritional basis, supplementation with vitamin E can be very helpful in the control and management of hot flushes. Other helpful supplements can be a multi B group vitamin supplement, Tryptophan (for sweating and insomnia), antioxidant vitamins and vitamin C with bioflavanoids. These should be prescribed on an individual basis, taking your daily nutritional intake into account.
9. Wear clothing made of natural fibres, thus avoiding promotion of irritation and sweating. Especially wear cotton underwear.
10. Ensure that underwear is not too tight, especially avoid bras that are tight or ill-fitting. A recent American study suggests that tight bras actually may help to develop congestion and irritation of breast tissue. The researchers cross referenced and compared western women with cultures who traditionally do not wear breast support!
11. Get plenty of exercise. Brisk walking is very helpful. Exercise has been discovered to help balance oestrogen metabolism and prevent osteoporosis.

Let your food be your medicine and your medicine be your food. (Hippocrates)

Understanding Plant Hormones — (Phyto-Oestrogens)

Many plants that are a standard part of our day-to-day diet contain plant oestrogens. On a nutritional basis, for women with breast cancer, plant hormones, in balance with the nutrients that they are partnered with in nature, may be a helpful and unrecognised healing tool in the management of the illness. Foods containing natural substances in balance, certainly are preferable to having to take huge quantities of artificial vitamins and minerals. The use of fresh foods including freshly made fruit and vegetable juices seems to help enormously.

I have noticed, as have various oncologists and other medical people, that patients who are attending to their nutritional status in this way, often have a corresponding improvement in vitality, general wellbeing and importantly, have fewer complications with treatment side effects. In particular, women dealing with breast cancer seem to obtain exceptional results with their level of wellbeing, using these sensible dietary adjustments.

Many of the vegetables commonly recommended for cancer patients are those that are naturally high in plant hormones or phyto-oestrogens. These are present in leafy greens, where high levels of natural calcium also are to be found. If you have low oestrogen, plant oestrogen will boost the effects of oestrogen in the body. The good news, however, is that if your oestrogen levels are high, plant oestrogens can decrease the effects by the mechanism of binding plant oestrogens to oestrogen receptors in the body. That is as natural substances in small doses, these plants contain chemistry that can help the body to create a hormonal balance. The safety factor with plant oestrogens and other plant hormones makes them attractive for use, particularly in managing menopause.

"Pharma Fem," a product made by Pharma foods in Sydney, Australia, is an excellent product, herbally-based and is worth considering as a replacement for HRT, but do find a natural therapist who can prescribe it for you. In other parts of the world there are many traditional medicines which, like Pharma Fem, may help you through the menopause in a natural way. Wherever possible use the healing power of nature, combined with your inner wisdom to help your healing.

So there are natural oestrogens that are safe and in natural balance within food substances. Fortunately, herbalists such as myself, now have access to an enormous amount of scientific botanical research to draw on. But the thing I find to be most fascinating about this is that somehow, former practitioners of traditional herbal medicine, knew what would work for a patient and they had no access to modern scientific validation or methods. Probably trial and error was involved, but I suspect it was the use of intuitive wisdom. It is also interesting that a high proportion of these practitioners were wise women.

Further Recommended Reading:

1. *Women's Bodies, Women's Wisdom,* by Chris Northrup, M.D. (Pub. by Bantam.)

Chapter Twelve

Osteoporosis—Keeping the Structure

Osteoporosis is a condition involving loss of bone density and strength. Many people seem to believe that it is due to women's hormonal shifts, particularly around the time of menopause. The process of osteoporosis, however, begins way before this. Nutritional patterns set in our early life seem to affect our bone density status in later life. Many women today show signs of osteoporosis in their thirties, long before menopause.

I recently came across some alarming figures that stated one woman in four will develop osteoporosis. By comparison, the figures are that one man in every forty is affected. One in every two women over the age of seventy suffers osteoporitic fractures and one in ten of those suffering hip fractures will die soon after, according to the study. It concluded by saying that more women will die from the consequences of hip fractures than from cancer of the breast, cervix and uterus combined!

A diagnosis of osteoporosis can be confirmed by a bone density test called a DEXA scan. It can show up on X-ray, however, it will only be evident by this method if more than 25% of bone density is already lost. Most diagnoses are made when bones have become so fragile that they can fracture very easily.

The usual approach to the management of osteoporosis is to increase calcium intake as well as to supplement with oestrogen (as in HRT). As a natural health therapist I would like to give you some information about osteoporosis and its development to provide a clearer picture of its management and prevention. Basically, as we examine all the relevant factors we begin to realise that osteoporosis is another lifestyle condition.

While calcium's role in osteoporosis is important, it is only a part of the whole story. Many factors contribute to why some women are more likely to suffer calcium loss than others. Supplementing with calcium alone will not be enough to correct the condition, let alone prevent it.

Firstly, there are a wide variety of illnesses that are involved with calcium loss in the body. It would therefore be imperative that these conditions be ruled out, otherwise any calcium supplementation you are taking is not likely to be utilised properly. A list of these conditions is as follows:

> anorexia, adrenal exhaustion, chronic digestive problems, (including absorption problems), Cushings disease, chronic alcoholism, diabetes and other blood sugar problems, steroid therapy, kidney disease, diseases of the thyroid gland and para-thyroid gland, leukaemia, liver disease and hormonal problems including early menopause.

What a list! As you can see from this large list of illnesses and conditions associated with calcium deficiency or malabsorption, it is a complex situation.

I believe it is useful to understand the nature of osteoporosis because once we are aware of the importance of lifestyle factors in helping to create this condition, we are obviously more empowered to do something positive about it.

I have been piecing together information over many years and I am pleased to see that the conclusions I have come to are being acknowledged now in journals of nutrition around the world. While replacing calcium in the diet and using oestrogen to slow down bone loss may be useful, clearly there are other important factors that need to be considered. Let us begin, however, by having a look at how calcium and oestrogen play their part in the story of osteoporosis.

Calcium

Bone contains the majority of the body's calcium, but it is a vital element in many other bodily functions. The bones themselves are dynamic tissues. They are not static—there is a continual balance going on between bone building and bone remodelling. The bones even act somewhat like a calcium storehouse which the other body processes can draw upon. Calcium can be withdrawn from the bone tissue into the bloodstream if there are not adequate supplies available to carry out essential body functions. The blood must maintain a constant level of calcium, as it is involved in maintaining the regularity of our heartbeat and the stimulation of our muscles. Calcium is also essential for the normal function of our brain and the process of digestion. If the bloodstream has been depleted of calcium by these other functions, it must quickly recover its balance. As this is imperative to our survival, calcium is withdrawn from our bones. Our para-thyroid glands play a major functional role here, ensuring that an adequate supply of calcium is available for blood stability.

It is important too that our digestive processes are working well. While calcium is primarily digested in the duodenum, its absorption and utilisation are directly affected by the body's levels of vitamin D, cortisol and oestrogen. Often, women approaching middle age begin to lose some of their digestive enzyme capabilities and stomach acid often can be low. This will alter the absorption or useability of the calcium they eat. It is thought that levels of stomach acid can be reduced by the ageing process, diets that have previously been excessively high in animal protein and overconsumption of antacid supplements.

Calcium From Food Sources

The consumption of dairy foods is being promoted heavily in many areas of society as the answer to osteoporosis. Heavy protein consumption has been related to this condition for many years in nutritional circles, but it seems to be overshadowed by the calcium theory. Dairy products contain protein, in fact skim milk products contain twice the protein content of whole milk products.

A study reported in The American Journal of Clinical Nutrition (1985) where researchers supplemented women's diets with 300mls of skim milk, three times daily, had an interesting and surprising outcome. The study was conducted over 12 months with 22 postmenopausal women. The amount of calcium that these women were receiving in the milk was 1500mg. Despite such high levels of calcium intake, these women were found to have no significant improvement! In summarising their report, the researchers concluded that the increase in protein intake, due to its high content in skim milk, attributed to their results. The 30% increase in protein was thought to cause calcium to be excreted via the kidneys. Presumably these women would have been consuming a standard American diet which is high in protein and high in fat. Therefore be cautious with the over-use of dairy foods, particularly if you have a diet high in protein already.

The far healthier option for adult women, and particularly women dealing with breast cancer, is to adopt a vegetarian way of eating for the period of your recovery. This will help balance oestrogen levels and maintain better bone integrity. If you go back to eating meats when you are well, have them as the condiment to a vegetable based meal, rather than the main course. I find that many women stay on a vegetarian diet with some small amounts of fish and free-range chicken after their recovery. In light of this knowledge of osteoporosis, and also the fact that vegetarian women have healthier oestrogen levels, this is indeed an attractive dietary package!

In studies of vegetarians and religious groups where vegetarian food is a way of life, we find some interesting facts about their differences in bone loss. These women show better bone density in their seventies as compared with meat eaters in their fifties. This is thought to be due to a lowered intake of protein.

On the other hand, it is known that eskimos consume more than 2000mg of calcium daily, and yet, as a group, they have one of the highest osteoporosis levels in the world. It is thought that their diet, which is incredibly high in protein, is the cause of the condition.

Women on a vegetarian diet can obtain large amounts of calcium from leafy green vegetables including broccoli, kale, mustard greens, seaweeds, legumes (beans and bean products.) Other excellent sources are chick peas, fresh tahini made from sesame seeds, fresh nuts, whole grains and bean curd, also known as tofu. If you add some ricotta cheese, cottage cheese and yoghurt to your diet as well you are looking at a very adequate calcium intake. Remember that adding a moderate amount of dairy products to your daily diet is far better if your protein intake is on the low to moderate side.

Sodium chloride

Sodium chloride is common salt. When added to food it too can interfere with the absorption of calcium in the body. Most people have excessive amounts of salt in their diet and benefit from reducing their intake. With rare exception, you will obtain quite enough salt in the food you eat. There is no need to add salt in cooking or at the table. Reducing your salt intake in this way will preserve calcium in the body that would otherwise be flushed out via the kidneys.

Calcium supplements

It would appear from research that apart from calcium that is naturally obtained in the diet, there are some supplemental forms of calcium that are better absorbed than others. Calcium as calcium orotate or as calcium citrate are two such forms. If you are having treatments involving the use of cortico-steroids, a calcium supplement is essential. Further, these calcium supplements should always be taken as a part of a complex, not just on their own. A high intake of a calcium on its own can lead to a deficiency of other minerals, for example magnesium, which can lead to heart problems and palpitations.

Other important minerals involved in bone health are the elements boron, silica, fluorine, phosphorus and magnesium. Boron has been of particular interest as it has recently been found to promote a potent form of oestrogen known as 17 beta estradiol. By a happy and rather remarkable "coincidence," all these minerals are found in nature in the right amounts and combinations with calcium-rich foods. A particularly good example of this is the leafy green vegetables.

Natural laws of botanical medicine like this are particularly useful when considering how to manage osteoporosis and what supplements may be worth taking. Other botanical principles to guide you are:

- Do not overdose on any one substance or you risk creating an imbalance.
- Overdosing will create the opposite reaction in the same part of the body that you were trying to heal. For example, high amounts of calcium taken on its own can lead to low magnesium levels. Low magnesium levels then lead to a reduction in bone mineralization. You were taking the calcium to help bone; but the result was that the excess calcium hindered bone formation.
- All things in moderation.

The message—loud and clear with all of this—is that dietary adjustments are the key ones that will make the difference. Herbal medicines contain natural plant material with the ingredients in balance. Herbal remedies are simply concentrated nutrition so their addition to your diet, instead of artificial substances, is my preference. As a herbalist it is good to know that nature has put together all these substances in their right partnerships and that my herbal mixtures are based on natural balance.

Oestrogen

Oestrogen has a place in the osteoporosis puzzle. It helps absorb calcium and preserve stores of collagen, while oestrogen receptors are found in bone. Although oestrogen does not have the ability to rebuild damaged bone it can help halt further bone loss.

As we have stated, bone is a dynamic, changing tissue. Its components are changing all the time. Menopause with its associated hormonal changes, particularly that of lowered amounts of oestrogen, affects the delivery of hormones to the bone structure. Bone turnover is a natural, inbuilt, erosive process which is carried out by cells called **osteoclasts.** This process is naturally balanced by another group of cells called **osteoblasts**. These cells contribute to the formation of new bone. Osteoclast activity is activated by oestrogen. Osteoblast activity is activated by progesterone.

These two components work hand in hand to keep bone erosion and bone remodelling in balance. So, in healthy bone tissue, the amount of bone removed by **osteoclast** activity is replaced by an equal amount of bone through **osteoblast** activity.

Changing hormonal levels can effect this erosion and remodelling process. We now know from many studies that there are strong suggestions our nutrition directly affects how oestrogen is produced and utilised in the body. It does seem that vegetarian women have lower blood levels of oestrogen than women who eat meat. Remember too that many plants contain phyto-oestrogens, and naturally these vegetarian women would have a high consumption of these foods which would help to keep oestrogens in the body in balance.

Vitamin D is best known for its roles in regulating calcium and bone formation. Another of oestrogen's functions is to activate vitamin D in the body. These two compounds then are involved in complex chemical reactions in the liver which reduce levels of free cortisol in the bloodstream. Cortisol is one of the hormones produced during the stress cycle and in excess it affects the immune system negatively. It also causes the resorption of bone. Treatments involving the use of cortisone and other steroid therapies have the same effects as do naturally high cortisol levels. These effects can directly aggravate or even produce osteoporosis. Therefore the combined effect of oestrogen and vitamin D in lowering cortisol levels is to reduce the bone resorbing effects of this hormone.

Dr. Ainslie Meares, the psychiatrist who originally helped my husband Ian with his meditation practice, had a theory of why meditation worked so well in cancer patients. His theory has since been substantiated by many people working in the field of behavioural and mind–body medicine. It seems that excess cortisol is produced in the body when it is under constant stress and meditation practice has the ability to reduce blood cortisol levels. So again, reducing cortisol levels helps to prevent bone resorption and osteoporosis.

Summary

1. Daily exercise is essential for natural and healthy hormonal balance. Brisk walking is an excellent form of exercise. Be gentle with yourself and enjoy your exercise time. However, exercising to the point of over-exertion tips the balance in the opposite direction. Female athletes who exercise to the point of having no periods have a substantial risk of the early development of osteoporosis. This is because hormonal levels are upset and there is often a depletion in progesterone.

2. If you are concerned about osteoporosis, have a thorough checkup and, if warranted, a DEXA scan. It is advisable to be checked for any of the illnesses that lead to calcium problems. These were listed at the beginning of this chapter.
3. Reduce the protein content of your diet. The high phosphate content of animal proteins helps calcium to be excreted via the kidneys. Excess intake of animal products should be avoided and replaced with a diet high in vegetables and fruits with grains, legumes and a small amount of easily-digested dairy foods such as natural yoghurt, cottage and ricotta cheese. Fish occasionally is recommended for many women.
4. Work towards lowering added salt in your diet especially pure sodium chloride. Sea salt, purchased as cubes and slightly darker in colour, is a better substitute if you need it. Salt requirement seems to be a very individual thing. Learn to enjoy the natural taste of foods and save your calcium, which can be excreted from the body in large amounts via the kidneys if you are a heavy salt user.
5. Coffee, sugar and alcohol are best eliminated from your diet, particularly if you have osteoporosis already. This makes good sense when we consider prevention from a general point of view.
6. A trip to see a natural therapist is advisable if you feel you may require gastric acid supplements. These MUST be prescribed for you. Research indicates that a high proportion of postmenopausal women (about 40%) are thought to be deficient in gastric acid secretions. This deficiency will hinder absorption of important minerals. Often, low stomach acid is indicated by chronic bad breath, bloating or indigestion after a protein meal. This condition can also be diagnosed by a capable Iridologist.

7. Use natural foods as much as possible as a part of your healing program. Use supplements wisely and only take the ones that have been prescribed for you. However, if you are taking oestrogen replacement or some prescribed medical drugs, vitamin and mineral supplements may be essential. Vitamin A, multi B complex supplement, vitamin C with Bioflavanoids and zinc are seen by many natural therapists as essential if you are taking HRT.
8. Stress management is an essential in the prevention and management of osteoporosis. Meditation practice is recommended highly for all. You may like to add to this with walking, Tai Chi, Yoga or Chi Kung. All these things will combine to make a better way of life.

Further Recommended Reading:

1. *Udder Nonsense: Why Cow's Milk is no Longer Required or Recommended*, by Nathaniel Mead and Martha C. Cottrell (to be published 1995, Avery Publishing Group, N.Y.)

Chapter Thirteen

Dealing With the Medical Issues Surrounding Breast Cancer

Diagnosis—Becoming Aware of your Emotional Anatomy

We have discussed previously, how women frequently have an intuitive knowing prior to their diagnosis—a sense that something within is "not right." It is as if there is an incubation period during which a woman is likely to be aware of subtle changes in her body and her hormonal fluctuations. I believe, as do many of my patients, that this is an attempt by the body to communicate to the mind. It is as if the undernurtured body was saying, "Remember me, I am down here, listen to me. I am tired and worn and I need attention!" Most of these women had a sense of the importance of these messages, but through force of circumstances, chose to ignore them. It was not until the time of diagnosis that the memory of this warning surfaced.

Often, during this "incubation" time of the illness, there are no physical symptoms present, just a vague feeling or awareness of changes in the body. Obviously these changes are too subtle for the equipment and diagnostic techniques of orthodox medicine to detect. Even with current technology, a tumour needs to be of reasonable size before it can be found. Also many pathology tests require substantial dysfunction before problems can be discovered.

I have come to understand through personal experience as well as from patient feedback, that a woman's entire reproductive system can be likened to a series of resonators or emotional barometers, measuring her state of being. Hormones, like the moisture in the air, cause the barometer to change—to rise or fall. Women notice these sensations in the body, but often do not realise the significance of them. Very often an area that is affected by cancer may have been giving warnings for a number of years. Some women have identified these areas as feeling like weak spots in the body or places where they have felt intermittent pain or discomfort for a long time.

In Ian's case, for many years he had noticed that his right leg had a chronic weakness in the mid thigh. This is where he eventually developed his cancer. Maybe in years to come, such patient observations may be able to be translated into earlier diagnosis. It is warranted to seek advice for such symptoms rather than ignore them. A doctor who specialises in preventative medicine and/or counselling, or a competent natural therapist, will be the best person to consult. Be aware too, that women can learn to read their own emotional barometer and need to learn to trust in what it is telling them.

Hopefully, many women will read this book with a view to the prevention of breast cancer, realise the power of their body's wisdom and learn to interpret it. I would hope and recommend that this awareness will lead you to a feeling of empowerment, learning to believe in your "gut feeling" and your intuition. This will give you the confidence and the ability to take whatever action is required.

Hormonal messages, in particular, may be warning signs worth listening to and trusting in. If medical science cannot give you a reason for feeling "below par," try making some lifestyle changes yourself. Notice any difference after a short trial period. A visit to a natural therapist for a complete health appraisal may be another way of getting started.

Most women will know instinctively what issues or habits require change in their lives. However, often it is not until some symptoms, or another person we respect prompts us, that we are moved to take the action that is required.

Women with breast cancer will often identify key body areas, commonly the solar plexus and the rib cage, which act as the storehouse for emotional tension and suppressed feelings. Breathing exercises and gentle bodywork, gentle massage and aromatherapy can all help and are excellent to add to meditation practice as a means to releasing these tensions. This can restore a healthy awareness and feeling to those areas in need of healing.

Dealing with diagnosis

Diagnosis can be experienced by women in so many different ways. For some it may come as a relief as well as a shock. The manner in which women are told both their diagnosis and their prognosis can make an enormous difference to the overall management of the illness, as well as the outcome. With a diagnosis of cancer, the doctor can clearly set an atmosphere that will enable the patient to respond either with an attitude of challenge and a view to possible healing, or to give in to the perceived power and fear of cancer. This is a point where doctors hold the power of life and death in their hands.

Breast cancer so often is represented in a way that instils and breeds fear into the minds and hearts of women. This is not to take attention away from the seriousness of the illness. However, the power to wield the staff of *healing*—within a medical profession and a media who view breast cancer as some kind of female curse—with a negative outcome, is a tall order.

Let us face it, if you are diagnosed by a medical profession that believes your cancer has no known cause, but will involve you in disfiguring and aggressive treatments that are viewed purely as palliative, and if you are in a society whose basic belief system supports that view, the picture may not seem all that rosy!

But I believe that the community wields an even greater power, one that can change *en masse* the fear about this disease that has crept into the consciousness of Western man. For you see, I have a different view—one that supports people and believes in possibility thinking. Ignorance and fear of cancer give it power to destroy, whereas understanding, knowledge and trust in ourselves instils the power to heal.

I was at this same crossroad with my husband Ian, nearly twenty years ago. At that time I had an opportunity to look this so-called enemy of society squarely in the eye. When I did so, I found it not nearly so scary and powerful as many people seem to perceive it. Never having been one to be short on the power of faith anyway, I was not daunted by the standard belief system of society or the medical statistics which said that Ian would have only three to six months to live.

While some people have a natural positivity that carries them through difficult circumstances, many of the people I work with have needed to **learn** how to develop a more positive state of mind. They have succeeded in this and transformed their lives.

However, it is not uncommon, at the time of initial diagnosis, when patients are informed of their medical conditions and treatments, that all information is lost in an abyss of shock, confusion and bewilderment. How interesting it is that for these people, somewhere deep within, there is a listening ear that hears the word cancer, hears the word prognosis and then becomes deaf to any other information given. Many say that this no longer happens in cancer medicine. I disagree—I see it all the time. And the result is that it makes the patient despondent and their supporting partner angry.

What is needed by people who are feeling hopeless and helpless in the face of life-threatening illness, is to hear words that can heal, words that can engender hope. They need to be in an atmosphere conducive to the encouragement of faith.

While it is quite possible to create this atmosphere in a caring medical setting, many patients complain of being affected by an overwhelming sense of medical doom and gloom. To be given a sentence or prognosis which involves the patient taking on a specific time limit for their life, almost always leads to a punctual appointment with death. If a patient takes this prognosis to a deep level within, I often feel powerless to help them to survive. Often, these people have lost their spirit, their will to live. Their belief system cannot accommodate possibility thinking or the will to heal. Instead of offering hope, the healing staff has dealt them a blow from which they may not recover. The best one can offer in this case is the possibility of a good death, for you see the patient can take on a definite prognosis like a negative affirmation, that takes hold as a part of the belief of the person. For these people, the belief system on their inside matches the belief system of the society outside. For them the word cancer fulfils and takes its place according to the belief system or consciousness of the wider community. For this group, cancer is simply a disease that kills. This is powerful stuff! Importantly, natural survivors operate with a different belief system. We can all learn from this and develop our own effective survival skills.

Maybe prognosis time could be an appropriate moment to access any skills of denial or ignorance that you have acquired! The following series of short true stories, will give you an understanding of how this works in practice.

Our first story is an incredible one, demonstrating the healing abilities of the mind–body connection and the power of a patient's belief system.

> An American "hill-billy" was diagnosed with throat cancer by his General Practitioner who told him that he would have to go to a large city hospital in order to have the cancer treated. The doctor also told him that this hospital had a new form of ray treatment that would cure his cancer. The man was

awed by the large hospital and after arrival there, was given a basic check up. When a thermometer was placed in this naive man's mouth, his doctor realised that the man thought that it was his ray treatment! After several sessions of this "wonder treatment" the man was cured—his cancer disappeared completely!

The next two stories powerfully demonstrate how belief systems can either turn on or turn off the *will to live.* These were both recorded by medical physiologist Walton Cannon. From his diary he states:

> Dr. S. M. Lambert of the Western Pacific Health Service of the Rockefeller Foundation wrote to me on several occasions he had seen evidence of death from fear. In one case there was a startling recovery.
>
> At a mission at Mona Mona in North Queensland were many native converts, but on the outskirts of the mission was a group of non-converts, including one Nebo, a famous witch doctor. The chief helper of the missionary was Rob, a native who had been converted. When Dr. Lambert arrived at the Mission he learned that Rob was in distress and that the missionary wanted him examined. Dr. Lambert made the examination, and found no fever, no complaint of pain, no symptoms or signs of disease. He was impressed, however, by the obvious indications that Rob was seriously ill and extremely weak. From the missionary he learned that Rob had had a *bone pointed* at him by Nebo and was convinced that, in consequence, he must die. Thereupon, Dr. Lambert and the missionary went for Nebo, threatened him sharply that his supply of food would be shut off if anything happened to Rob and that he and his people would be driven away from the mis-

> sion. At once Nebo agreed to go with them to see Rob. He leaned over Rob's bed and told the sick man that it was all a mistake, a mere joke—indeed, that he had not pointed a bone at all.
>
> The relief, Dr. Lambert testifies, was almost instantaneous. That evening Rob was back at work, quite happy again and in full possession of his physical strength.

A less fortunate outcome is reported in the next account.

> Dr. Lambert wrote to me concerning an experience of Dr. P. S. Clarke with Kanakas working on the sugar plantations of North Queensland.
>
> One day a Kanaka came to his hospital and told him he would die in a few days because a spell had been put upon him and nothing could be done to counteract it. The man had been known by Dr. Clarke for some time. He was given a very thorough examination, including an examination of the stool and urine. All was found normal, but as he lay in bed he gradually grew weaker. Dr. Clarke called upon the foreman of the Kanakas to come to the hospital to give the man assurance, but on reaching the foot of the bed, the foreman leaned over, looked at the patient, and then turned to Dr. Clarke, saying, "Yes, doctor, close up him he die." (i.e., he is nearly dead). The next day, at 11 o'clock in the morning, he ceased to live.

Compare the technique used in the last two stories with our hill-billy friend in the first story. The first story gives a positive message to the patient of **hope** of a cure and then he is provided with a technique and a ritual by which the cure can happen (i.e. the use of the thermometer). Whereas in our other two stories, due to the belief systems of the tribe which dictates that if you are "pointed" with a bone by the witch doctor, you die. While hope is removed and a strong belief and expectation that death will result exists in the mind of the patient, in reality it becomes a self-fulfilling prophesy.

Bone Pointing or the Negative Placebo: The Story That Does Not Heal

Just as someone can create a story with images of a life-affirming nature, so they can tell us a negative story that, according to what our belief system is, potentially has the power to enter our consciousness, find its way to the spirit or soul nature, and extinguish the spark of life—the will to live. Such is the nature of *bone pointing* or the negative placebo response, as it is known in behavioural medicine. I have personally witnessed this power of belief as related to healing in many other cultures throughout the world, as well as in the context of orthodox medical practise.

Australian aboriginal society has a code of ethical conduct, which, if transgressed in a serious manner, may result in being "pointed." One is pointed at with a long human bone by the medicine man or kadaitja man, as he is known in Central Australia. He is a man of high degree, capable of strong thought powers. The person who is pointed knows once this has happened, he is as good as dead. He is then shunned by all and will not be able to cope, becoming hopeless, losing all expectation of help from any outside source. With his social structure destroyed, he waits for death. Just prior to death, the tribe gather to say good-bye and he dies.

The cancer story, I believe, is a more modern-day ritual, similar in many ways to bone pointing. In cancer, belief systems and strong thoughts about disease have the power to be life-giving or destroying—the difference being, that somehow in Western society, we have forgotten about the power of healing through using a patient's own belief system as well as ritual.

For the medical profession it is now a matter of choosing how to tell the story, and for the patient, it is a matter of choice whether they wish to accept it or not. There is an obvious need for honesty, clarity and directness at diagnosis time, but not at the sacrifice of the subtle but important life qualities like hope, faith, and love. There are things in our lives that we cannot quantify through science, that make the livingness of life throb with the passion to be. If medicine fails to provide sustenance to feed the will to live, it is lacking in one of the most crucial elements in healing. Spirit, thought and belief need to take their rightful place again in medicine.

Currently medicine has an emphasis on treating rather than healing. Each has its part to play in caring for the patient, but it is the fusion of the two that will lead to a better way of living and a medicine that serves its people.

How Women React Emotionally to Diagnosis

A difficult time for patients and their partners around the time of diagnosis is usual. This is an experience that no one can prepare either of you for. The best that everyone can do, however, is to be honest with feelings and emotions. Often, great understanding and compassion is required as there may be unfamiliar emotions demonstrated, especially in the company of family and friends. For, while a patient may appear passive with medical helpers, some women will rediscover their feelings with great intensity, discharging them in the safety of the home environment.

Mood swings can be of some concern, but it is far better to allow yourself the luxury to **really feel** how you feel for maybe even a week or two. Some women can move through and express moods of grief, shock, denial, anger, or resentment, and may even find themselves bargaining for time with God in their private prayer moments. These reactions to diagnosis are stages of grief that are quite similar to the stages of dying that Dr. Elisabeth Kubler-Ross talks about in her classic "*Death and Dying.*" They are also normal.

However, for some, the process can be more protracted. Some women will cope well enough on their own, while others will benefit from outside help. It can be quite an individual experience, however, depending on many factors.

Taking this individuality into consideration is so important in helping the patient find what is best for them to do. I could see six patients in the one day, all with the same type of breast cancer, but by understanding their individuality and listening to their story, finding out who they are, it allows them to move into territory that is much deeper than their symptoms present. Del's and Betty's stories highlight just how different people can be in coping with their breast cancer diagnosis.

Del's Story

I remember Del as one who reacted and coped in her own rather independent way. Best described as a rather crusty woman, she had been brought up in the bush where her dad had practised as a G.P. With her dry wit and a steely exterior, she had the appearance of a woman who had just stepped out of a Crocodile Dundee movie set! I really liked her earthiness and enjoyed visiting her at home.

She had, as she expressed it, "Taken a lot of knocks in her life," and she was indeed a strong and independent woman, who kept to herself. Apart from her two old dogs and a small herd of milking goats, she lived alone. She really loved the old dogs that she introduced to me on my first visit as the world's best counsellors, because they said nothing and gave lots of love! I took that comment as a strong hint!

She had been diagnosed with breast cancer and saw no difficulty with the idea of a mastectomy. Well, she said dryly. "What do I need them for, and I'm past the "change?" I told the doctor to just get rid of the damn thing (the breast). Can't let a little thing like that interfere with my life can I?" I was unusually lost for words!

Del had recovered quickly from her surgery and refused any further treatment as she said she had a total belief that it would fix her. Her dad had been a great believer in surgery, she told me. This cancer was not going to slow her down and, after all, she had just bought herself a new chainsaw before diagnosis, and she was keen try it out! "You know, I reckon I just let myself get a bit down over things. My brother Jack died last year, the last of my relatives. Knocked me a bit, it did. I guess I just got to get on with life, I'm not ready to meet my maker yet!"

Del fully believed that ridding herself of her diseased breast would fully cure her. It did. She lived on for another twenty years in good health and died from a heart attack due to over-exertion. In all the time I knew Del, I never once offered her advice. I would simply sit and have a cup of tea, buy my goats' milk, listen and leave. Although her exterior was weathered, I remember that Del had a heart of gold and a feminine strength that I can instantly recall to this day. Definitely not the chiffon type of femininity, but the real deep, old magic of the wise woman. I learned much from her.

Betty's Story

Betty, on the other hand, was a lady in the true sense of the word. Unlike Del, she had been very particular and proud of her appearance, and always presented herself in a manner that highlighted her attractiveness. Also a perfectionist by nature, the effect of the removal of one breast was devastating to the whole structure of her life.

After diagnosis, without being given the time to comprehend or psychologically adapt to life with one breast, Betty was scheduled for surgery within days, due to a "fortunate" cancellation. She underwent a mastectomy, without having any advice on reconstruction, counselling or advice about what might happen later. Betty had quite large breasts and the lack of one of them, physically caused a severe balance problem as well as tremendous difficulties with self esteem and appearance. After surgery, both Betty and her husband were stunned and could not communicate easily with any of the medical staff.

Sadly, but not surprisingly, Betty suffered post-surgical depression—and I mean **suffered,** in the true sense of the word. Eventually shock therapy was recommended as the treatment of choice, and for a while it did snap her out of her depressed state. Although this helped Betty to be functional on a day-to-day basis, her inner self retreated more and more.

A few years later I saw Betty and her husband again when she had been diagnosed with bone secondaries. It had been her husband's decision to come and see me and I was shocked to see a woman whose outer presence was quite strong, but whose inner life was clearly clouded behind distant and disconnected eyes. I had read of the Shaman practice of soul retrieval, and could think of no other accurate image to portray how much of this woman's spirit was missing.

It took about half an hour into the conversation before I felt any reconnection with Betty at all. Her passive exterior, seemingly covered over the fierceness of her pain. But with wise counsel, that is encouraging her to talk, and me to listen with my heart, she began to move forward and made a major decision to rekindle the spark of life and retrieve, piece by piece, the missing links in her life.

Unlike Del, who was glad to see the tail end of her breast, it was not so for Betty. Such is the uniqueness of each person's journey.

As the story unfolded, Betty had not ever been able to grieve for her missing breast, and she confided in me that she had been unable to look at her body in a mirror since the surgery. Rather than taking showers, she would take bubble baths that would hide the disfigurement from view. In conversation she often referred to her mastectomy site as "the scene of the crime." Her husband was an incredibly dedicated and committed man who supported Betty through the most terrible times, and never gave up hope of retrieving his wife back from a void that he could neither see nor understand. This story has been ten years in the making and so far Betty continues towards emotional healing. She is currently enthusiastically investigating the possibility of a breast reconstruction.

What Patients Want from their Doctors and from the Medical Profession in General

I believe that the orthodox medical system, the complementary medical system, and all of the naturopathic healing systems, should be service-oriented and user-friendly. Our organisation obtains much feedback about how their doctors are looking after them. Most patients actually enjoy comparing and sharing their information and experiences. The following information was gathered as a result of surveys conducted during The Gawler Foundation's groups and this paper was presented by Ian at The Royal College of General Practitioners Annual Conference in 1991. An audio tape of this presentation is available from The Gawler Foundation as tape number 14.

Patients and their Doctors—What works?

The Patients' View: Where the Medical System is Being Effective in Cancer Management

1. Technical Skills:
    - Diagnosis and Referral
    - Surgery
    - Buying time in some cases and extending life
    - Relieving symptoms and treating pain.
2. Communication Skills/Humanity:
    - Compassion
    - Providing a sense of security and comfort in the system
    - Responding to patient's requests.

The Patients' View: Where the Medical System Provides Ineffective Management

1. Technical Skills:
   - Delayed diagnosis, ineffective diagnosis
   - Poor clinical judgement
   - Dismissing reported symptoms
   - Through over-familiarity, becoming too casual with symptoms/patient
   - Having a lack of time
   - Poorly matched referrals (in personal sense)
   - Unable to communicate at patient's level.
2. Communication Skills:
   - Removing hope, pointing of the bone!
   - Poor communication generally
   - Holier than thou attitude:
     - intellectual superiority
     - nondisclosure of information
     - resent questioning and get angry when asked about options
     - professional or personal ego problems
   - "Difficult patient" syndrome.
3. Attitudes:
   - Closed mind — barrier to the non-scientific
   - Tunnel vision—the impact of specialisation
   - Treat the disease and overlook, or avoid, the person
   - Lack of knowledge and/or acceptance of self-help techniques
   - Dismiss as "alternative nonsense" the right to have a choice—including natural and complementary therapies.

What Patients Ask of Their Doctors:

1. We want ACCESS to:
    - The best available medical treatment.
    - The best available self-help techniques.
2. Be a good communicator:
    - Provide information—your truth
        - Underpinned with hope
        - Use statistics, keep open-ended
        - Advise on all options
        - Advise on lifestyle issues after first treatment to avoid secondaries
        - Use language I can understand
        - Answer questions
    - Be positive
    - Use active listening skills
    - Give time—be available
        - for appointments (long as arranged)
        - after hours—in emergency
        - reassurance takes time!
3. Treat me as a person, not just a disease.
4. Provide ongoing support regardless of my choices.
5. Be a PARTNER—SOMEONE I CAN TRUST!

Patients' Suggestions to Improve Communication

1. Understand I may not be acting normally.
2. Sit close to me and avoid barriers (e.g. desks)
3. Please touch me
    - handshakes

- arm on shoulder
- hug, if congruent

4. Use eye contact
5. Listen to me
   - acknowledge what you hear
   - seek confirmation that your messages are heard
   - use educational aids including handouts
   - reinforce what you say frequently.
6. Recommend partners attend consultations
7. Advise taking notes or taping major consultations.
8. Respect my feelings, beliefs and hopes
9. Take an interest in my family.

A Patient's Statement:

Do not feel that you have failed if you treat me well and I do not recover.

Be at peace with death.

Doctors treat, God cures.

Understand my need for you to be infallible; I would prefer you to have a magic wand, but I will understand if you respect that desire, are patient and aren't.

Further Recommended Reading:

1. *Breast Cancer: The Complete Guide*, by Yashan Hirshaut, M.D., F.A.C.P. and Peter I. Pressman, M.D., F.A.C.S. (Pub. by Bantam.)
2. *Love Medicine and Miracles*, by Bernie Siegal, M.D. (Pub. by Harper Perennial.)

Chapter Fourteen

Breast Cancer: Who is Responsible?

Currently, breast cancer is a topical issue in the western world. Consequently it is also the subject of much political banter.

From my point of view, as a woman and mother of four, combined with my experience, I am led to believe that we, as women, need to be the ones to own our bodies. We are the ones who need to take responsibility for how we live our lives and for how we heal our lives. We are responsible.

Life gives us an opportunity to respond to this challenge of personal responsibility as well as to find out how we, as women, can contribute to the whole. In doing so, not only do we heal ourselves, but we begin to take responsibility on a planetary scale. Women innately know this. They know it in their hearts and their souls, but for some reason feel devalued in a patriarchal society and so often they are limited in doing something about it. Often they feel powerless to act. Powerless to bring forth the changes that they perceive are needed to make this a better world to live in.

Our planet Earth is also ill. She too, The Earth Mother, has the early signs of breast cancer and is in need of healing. Her circulation, her blood (the rivers) are toxic and polluted, her lungs (the trees) are being destroyed, her skin (the crust) is manifest with a pox caused by the ravages of war, nuclear explosions and the excessive delving into her depths to steal her treasure.

As women, we wield commercial power, for we are the consumers of society. We buy the medicine, the goods, the food.

What we choose to buy can make a difference. What we choose to think can make a difference. How we choose to be can make a difference.

Mothers of the future generations can learn—learn that it is not politics and more scientific paraphernalia that will heal—it is ultimately ourselves. Waking up to the power of our own consciousness; taking back our true feminine power; transforming our devaluedness into strength and truth; then we can be responsible for shaping our health and shaping the future.

It is not our government or our hospital system that we should be blaming for the apathy shown towards the breast cancer issue. Surely we, as women, have some responsibility towards the care for the bodies we inhabit. Public and community organisations may be responsible for the aftercare of patients, but are they responsible for the detection and cause of our own illnesses? I think not. Maybe it hurts, maybe it is a bitter pill to swallow, but is it not easier to blame the outside world for what is going wrong in our lives! Maybe if we were honest with ourselves, it is within ourselves that we should be looking to find these answers.

People need people. Science may cure us temporarily, but can it heal the very essence of our being—the Pandora's box of emotions, thoughts and concerns of the spirit where our disharmonies dwell? Women's conflict in reality is to do with keeping the balance between spirit and matter, psyche and body. Our conflicts are also about isolation, devaluation, social and community issues. We all walk the soil of this earth and eventually we all go back to it. We are all connected and yet we are all so far apart. We have incredible communication systems that network across the globe and yet we do not communicate well with those close to us. Sometimes we do not even know the names of our neighbours. How strange for a society that not all that many years ago, was living in communal villages. Now, more than ever, we are required to utilise that wonderful, nurturing energy in a positive and life enhancing way. Community spirit needs to find its way into our hearts again. Every woman needs to feel, to have a sense of feminine connectedness, for that is the very thread of the fabric of our life. Only then will we have an edge on issues such as breast cancer and other inherent health problems.

We have an opportunity to respond to all these issues in a way that will increase our personal awareness and empowerment.

Part Three

Appendices

APPENDIX I
BREAST CANCER—SOME KEY REFERENCES

ARTICLE 1: Psychological Identification of Breast Cancer Patients Before Biopsy

(*J. Psychosom. Res.*, Vol. 26, No. 1, pp. 1–10, 1982)
By Michael Wirsching, *et al.*

Abstract—Fifty-six women admitted consecutively for a breast biopsy were interviewed on the day prior to the operation. Interviewer ratings and blind ratings (audiotapes) allowed a [statistically significant (a = 5%)] differentiation of women in whom the biopsy revealed a cancer from those whose tumor was benign. The ratings took into account characteristics assumed to be typical of the women with cancer: (1) being inaccessible or overwhelmed when interviewed; (2) emotional suppression with sudden outbursts; (3) rationalization; (4) little or no anxiety before the operation; (5) demonstration of optimism; (6) superautonomous self-sufficiency; (7) altruistic behaviour; (8) harmonization and avoidance of conflicts. On the basis of the interviews the interviewer and a blind rater predicted the correct diagnosis in 83% and 94% of all cancer patients and in 71% and 68% of all benign cases. This result is also significant (a = 5%).

The identified psychological syndrome was found in all breast cancer patients but also in a quarter to a third of the patients with benign nodes. We interpret it as a long-standing defensive pattern adopted in the face of extreme emotional stress. A possible etiological significance for the cancerous disease cannot be derived from this study.

ARTICLE 2: Influence of Physician Communication on Newly Diagnosed Breast Patients' Psychologic Adjustment and Decision-Making

(Reproduced in *Cancer* 1994, 74:336–341)
By Cleora S. Roberts, PhD., Charles E. Cox, M.D., Douglas S. Reintgen, M.D., Walter E. Baile, M.D., and Michael Gibertini, PhD.

Background—Physician-patient communication is of critical importance when a breast cancer diagnosis is made, because the emotionally overwhelmed patient must be educated about her disease and available treatments so she can participate in decisions about her care. A research study addressed the hypothesis that patients whose surgeons used psychotherapeutic techniques during the cancer diagnostic interview would have better psychologic adjustment to their cancer.

Conclusions—Provision of information needed for decision-making appears to be valued largely within the context of a caring physician-patient relationship. Specific surgeons' behaviour believed to facilitate patient adjustment include expressing empathy, allowing sufficient time for patients to absorb the cancer diagnosis, providing information and engaging the patient in treatment decision-making.

ARTICLE 3: A Breast Cancer Support Group: Activities and Value to Mastectomy Patients

(*Group Support,* 1993)
By Betty Satterwhite Stevenson, MA and Patricia M. Coles, MS

Abstract—This study surveys the reasons women attend a breast cancer support group as well as the perceived benefits of attending one. The hope of receiving and giving emotional support and of obtaining increased information were the largest single factors in attendance. Our results indicate that these hopes are realized. Patients should be offered the opportunity to attend support groups, as they provide added and needed assistance, especially in the areas of new information on cancer and coping with its psychosocial sequelae.

ARTICLE 4: Group Support for Patients with Metastatic Cancer

(*Arch. Gen. Psychiatry*, 1981, 38:527)
By David Spiegel, MD, *et al.*

The effects of weekly supportive group meetings for women with metastatic carcinoma of the breast were systematically evaluated in a one-year, randomized, prospective outcome study. The groups focused on the problems of terminal illness, including improving relationships with family, friends, and physicians and living as fully as possible in the face of death. We hypothesized that this intervention would lead to improved mood, coping strategies, and self-esteem among those in the treatment group. Eighty-six patients were tested at four-month intervals. The treatment group had significantly lower mood-disturbance scores on the Profile of Mood States scale, had fewer maladaptive coping responses, and were less phobic than the control group. This study provides objective evidence that a supportive group intervention for patients with metastatic cancer results in psychological benefit. Mechanisms underlying the effectiveness of this group intervention are explored.

ARTICLE 5: Effect of Psychosocial Treatment on Survival of Patients with Metastatic Breast Cancer

(*The Lancet*, 1989: p. 888)
By David Spiegel, *et al.*

Summary—The effect of psychosocial intervention on time of survival of 86 patients with metastatic breast cancer was studied prospectively. The 1 year intervention consisted of weekly supportive group therapy with self-hypnosis for pain. Both the treatment (n = 50) and control groups (n = 36) had routine oncological care. At 10 year follow-up, only 3 of the patients were alive, and death records were obtained for the other 83. Survival from time of randomisation and onset of intervention was a mean 36.6 (SD 37.6) months in the intervention group compared with 18.9 (10.8) months in the control group, a significant difference. Survival plots indicated that divergence in survival began at 20 months after entry, or 8 months after intervention ended.

Note: All the long term survivors did attend the group!

ARTICLE 6: Survival Hazards Analysis in First Recurrent Breast Cancer Patients: Seven-year Follow-up

(*Psychosom. Med.* 50:520–528 (1988))
By Sandra M. Levy, *et al.*

The purpose of this study was to identify predictors of survival time in first recurrent breast cancer patients, including psychologic as well as biologic factors. Beginning in 1979, 36 women being treated at the National Institutes of Health for histologically proven recurrent disease were enrolled in this prospective study. At the time of data analysis, 24 had died from their malignancy. Through the use of a Cox proportional hazards model, four factors significantly entered the equation predicting survival time in the sample: Patients with a longer disease-free interval who expressed more joy at baseline testing, who were predicted to live longer by their physicians, and who had fewer metastatic sites tended to live longer with recurrent disease than others in the sample. ($X^2 = 22.9$, $p < 0.0001$). Findings from recent clinical and animal studies suggest that regulatory systems within the organism are linked and potentially influence one another. This study has demonstrated that factors at a number of levels—behavioural, as well as biologic—need to be considered in accounting for disease outcome variance.

ARTICLE 7: Which Patients are Cured of Breast Cancer?

(*British Medical Journal*, Volume 289, 1984, 1108–1111)
By I. S. Fentiman, J. Cuzick, R. R. Millis, J. L. Hayward

Abstract—The clinical and pathological features of 51 patients who survived for more than 20 years after diagnosis of cancer of the breast were compared with those of 178 contemporaries who died within 20 years after diagnosis. Of those who survived, 18 (35%) had had pathologically affected axillary nodes compared with at least 86 (49%) of those who died. Also, 11 (21%) of the survivors had had small tumours compared with 10 (8%) of those who died. Pathological review of tumours in the survivors showed 40 (78%) to have been infiltrating ductal carcinomas, of which 13 (32%) were grade 3 lesions. These differences between the two groups were largely due to the prognostic value of these variables in the first five years after diagnosis. After a patient had survived five years the major prognostic variables were of little value in the prediction of which patients would be cured of breast cancer.

Age, menstrual state, clinical stage, and axillary nodes being affected are thus of some prognostic value in cancer of the breast, but the present inadequacy of knowledge of the behaviour of the disease makes accurate prediction of which patients will be cured impossible.

ARTICLE 8: Stress and Relapse of Breast Cancer

BMJ, Volume 298, February 1989, p. 291.
Amanda J. Ramirez, *et al.*

Abstract—To elucidate the association between stressful life events and the development of cancer the influence of life stress on relapse in operable breast cancer was examined in matched pairs of women in a case-control study. Adverse life events and difficulties occurring during the postoperative disease free interval were recorded in 50 women who had developed their first recurrence of operable breast cancer and during equivalent follow up times in 50 women with operable breast cancer in remission. The cases and controls were matched for the main physical and pathological factors known to be prognostic in breast cancer and sociodemographic variables that influence the frequency of life events and difficulties. Severely threatening life events and difficulties were significantly associated with the first recurrence of breast cancer. The relative risk of relapse associated with severe life events was 5.67 (95% confidence interval 1.57 to 37.20), and the relative risk associated with severe difficulties was 4.75 (1.58 to 19.20). Life events and difficulties not rated as severe were not related to relapse. Experiencing a non-severe life event was associated with a relative risk of 2.0 (0.62 to 7.47), and experiencing a non-severe difficulty was associated with a relative risk of 1.13 (0.38 to 3.35).

These results suggest a prognostic association between severe life stressors and recurrence of breast cancer, but a larger prospective study is needed for confirmation.

ARTICLE 9: Changes in the Investigation and Management of Primary Operable Breast Cancer in Victoria

(*Medical Journal of Australia,* Vol. 161, 18 July 1994, 110–120).
David J. Hill, Victoria M. White, Graham G. Giles, John P. Collins and Paul R. B. Kitchen

Objectives: To investigate the surgical practice and adjuvant therapies used in the treatment of primary operable breast cancer in Victoria in 1990 and compare them with results of a similar study in 1986.
Results: Most patients (82%) were referred to surgeons by general practitioners. Mammographic screening detected 14% of the cancers. The proportion of women receiving breast-conserving operations rose from 22% to 1986 to 42% in 1990. Surgeons operating on more than 20 breast cancers per annum were most likely to perform breast-conserving operations. The most common reasons given for non-conservative operations were the size of the tumour (37%), its central location (25%) and/or patient concern about the risk of recurrence if the breast was to be conserved (22%). Among these patients, reconstruction was done at the time of primary treatment in 13%, subsequently in 2%, and was planned by another 5%. Of all patients, 33% were referred to a radiation oncologist and 24% actually received radiotherapy (similar to 1986). Medical oncologists saw 33% of the patients and 20% of all patients who received chemotherapy (similar to in 1986), which was given by a medical oncologist in 83% of the cases. Use of endocrine therapy increased from 20% in 1986 to 40% in 1990.

ARTICLE 10: Changing Trends—An overview of Breast Cancer Incidence and Mortality

(Reproduced in *Cancer* 1994; 74:222–227).
Lawrence Garfunkel, M.A., Catherine C. Bering, M. P. H., and Clark W. Heath, Jr. M.D.

The incidence of breast cancer rose about 1% per year between 1940 and 1980 according to data in the Connecticut Tumor Registry. A sharp increase of 32% was reported between 1980 and 1987 in the Surveillance, Epidemiology and End Results Program of the National Cancer Institute. Data from this program shows that the increase in incidence was due to localized cases and cancers of less than 2 cm in greatest dimension. In addition, a sharp increase in carcinoma in situ was observed. The increase in breast cancer incidence coincides with an increased use of mammography in asymptomatic women in the 1980s. Mortality from breast cancer has changed little since the 1930s, but the increases in localized and small-size tumors and decreases in the rate of tumors of 3 cm or larger at diagnosis indicates that breast cancer mortality may start to decrease. Evidence from provisional breast cancer monthly mortality data suggests that there was a 3–5% drop in 1991 compared to 1990.

ARTICLE 11: Battling Breast Cancer with Dollars and Sense

(Editorial, Medical Journal of Australia, Vol. 161, 18 July 1994)
Alan Langlands, Chairman, Division of Radiation Oncology, Westmead Hospital.

It is almost impossible in 1994 in Australia to open a newspaper, read a magazine or watch an evening's television without breast cancer being discussed or appeals for research monies being made. The extent of this preoccupation with the disease is coming close to a form of medical hysteria.

The facts are now well known. Each year, over 6000 Australian women will be diagnosed with breast cancer and some 500 women will die from this disease. Such has been the force of this publicity that politicians are moving rapidly to provide more money, but with the debate regarding what should be done with that money—or whether needs are being addressed by its provision—coming *after* the nomination of the funds to be provided.

In this issue of the Journal, three more articles are added to the 3000 or so that are published each year. Many of the 3000 will present the results of "research"; many will repeat the impelling demand that "more research is needed".

It is perhaps time to stop and think. Some realism, if not fatalism, is creeping into the discussion. In spite of the hype which surrounds many of the publications and regular "breakthroughs" the fact remains that breast cancer is an incurable disease.[1] So much so that a recent editorial in *The Lancet* was entitled "Breast cancer: have we lost our way?".[2] It challenged clinicians and basic researchers to meet and try to find novel ways to approach this disease.

In a report of the subsequent meeting, the answer was an emphatic "No, we have not lost our way", but there was little to suggest where the new initiatives are coming from.[3] Much of the report deals with the problem of scientific fraud in clinical trials. Particular concern was expressed at the decision by the National Cancer Institute in the United States to suspend new patient recruitment to 14 studies. This is certainly a backward step, as these studies have been among the most important in making modest advances in the treatment of breast cancer. Nevertheless, it emphasises the increasing complexity of the structure and administration of clinical trials. The days of trials within single institutions are obviously over. On-site review of trial procedures by external experts will become the norm. Thus, clinical trials will become complex and difficult to carry out.[4]

At present, some advances in basic research make the care of patients with breast cancer more difficult. Translating the multitude of findings into guidelines for clinical management is a significant problem. What are clinicians to make of the 20-plus "potentially useful prognostic indicators" which have been identified as a result of basic research?[5] What is the value of a prognostic indicator in incurable disease?

Turning research into practice also strikes administrative barriers. For example, testing for hormone receptors, which are important in predetermining the response to some adjuvant therapies, still does not attract a Medicare benefit if done by immunocytochemical techniques—techniques which are essential for assessing the small tumours discovered by our screening programs.

Real breakthroughs in genetics occur almost daily. The breast cancer gene has been identified—no doubt it will be cloned and blood tests for its identification will become available. The huge dilemma facing us now is not only further research on the gene itself but determining what resources will be needed to make use of the information that it provides.

The ethics of testing unaffected men and women in kindreds where there is familial breast cancer needs to be discussed. Surely there is a dilemma in testing for a gene which is a marker for a disease at a time when it is considered to be incurable? Some would argue that these patients should be offered subcutaneous mastectomy, but do we know that subcutaneous mastectomy is effective? If we do, when should it be carried out? If we do not, what should we do? What clinical research should follow? Can we centralise data? What genetic counselling needs to be available? And, most of all, do we have these resources?

The answer is obviously "no". Do we have the planning processes and the foresight to see they are in place within the next few years, by which time the gene will have been cloned and tests will become commercially available? Again the answer is "no". The disaster which looms is the erratic introduction of genetic testing purely as a service to those who can afford to pay.

If the valuable research which has already been done is to do any good for women with breast cancer, significant resources are needed at the clinical interface. It is simplistic to assume that the funding of research without attention to its implications for patient management is the solution to the problem. How will we give effect to our burgeoning knowledge? *That* is the debate which must begin now.

References:

1. McKay, M., Langianda, A. O. Prognostic factors in breast cancer [letter]. *N. Engl. J. Med.* 1992, 327:1317–1318.
2. Breast cancer/have we lost our way? (editorial), *Lancet* 1993, 341:343–344.

3. Evans. The challenge of breast cancer. *Lancet* 1994, 343:1085–1088.
4. Breast cancer: clearing trails in the forest, without losing our way [editorial], *Lancet* 1994, 343:1049–1050.
5. National Cancer Institute. Potentially useful prognostic indicators in node-negative breast cancer. *J. Natl. Cancer Inst.* 1993, 85:1206–1219.

APPENDIX II
REFERENCES—MIND, IMMUNITY AND BREAST CANCER

1. Bageley, C. **Control of the emotions, remote stress, and the emergence of breast cancer.** *Indian. J. Clin. Psychol.* 6:213–220, 1979.

   113 women (aged less than 70 yrs) with early cancer were studied preoperatively; Subjects had been admitted to the hospital for breast tumor biopsy and had no apparent knowledge of the suspected diagnosis. After biopsies, comparisons of the 45 Subjects with cancer and the 68 with benign tumors revealed significant correlations between breast cancer and (a) the occurrence of subjectively stressful events (social, psychological, and physical) up to 15 yrs before appearance of a breast tumor, and (b) a chronic behavioural pattern of abnormal emotional expression, specifically, concealment of emotions and bottling up of anger.

2. Baltrusch H. J. **Problems, tasks and limits of psychosomatic cancer research.** *J. Psychosom. Med.* 9:285–294.

   ◆ psychotherapy

   The problem and tasks confronting psychosomatic cancer research are seen to fall into four major categories including psychological and psychophysiological investigations, psychosomatic animal research, and psychotherapy research in cancer. The effects of personality patterns on the development of cancer and its progress; definition of a "cancer prone personality"; affinity of certain types of malignancy to different personality types; evaluation of psychological states, such as despair and depression, as contributing factors; incidence of cancer in persons with abnormal or psychotic behaviour patterns; group investigations on a transcultural basis in different countries, civilizations and societies; investigation of the everyday habits of cancer patients with regard to eating, smoking, and drinking, etc.; and comparison of different age groups characterized by high cancer incidence, such as childhood and old age. As a second area of study on research studies on neurohormonal and immunologic functions, the role of chronic inflammations and trauma, and the previous history of the cancer patient with respect to psychosomatic background data are listed. As to the third area, psychosomatic animal experiments, it is advocated that such experiments be conducted in species "sociologically close" to man. In the fourth category, psychotherapy, it is speculated that if psychosocial factors are able to influence malignancy growth and its course, there are possibly also psychosocial factors which may strengthen the host defence of the organism. The role of psychotherapy in the overall treatment of cancer patients is discussed with regard to the reduction of anxiety and tension, the reinforcement of the patient's will to survive and to cope with life-threatening disease, as well as with regard to secondary prevention and rehabilitation.

3. Baltrusch, H.J.F., Waltz M. **Cancer from a biobehavioral and social epidemiological perspective.** *Soc. Sci. Med.* 20:789–794, 1985.

   ◆ behaviour modification

   Malignant neoplasms should not be viewed as a "psychogenic" nor as "primarily organic" disease but as an interaction of various forces, in which psychosocial factors may play an important role. To understand the increase in neoplastic disease which has taken place in this century requires a theoretical framework including social, psychosocial and behavioural dimensions, as well as the endocrine and immunologic mechanisms acting as pathogenic pathways. Recent theoretical developments in health psychology and allied disciplines on coping behaviour and social support should be integrated into biomedical models of the etiology, pathogenesis, and clinical course of malignant neoplasia. Environmental stressors, as well as mediating variables at the cognitive, affective, behavioural and physiological levels of adaptation, are suggested as major components of a model of multidimensional pathology. A growing body of research on the role of psychosocial factors in adjustment to cancer and its treatment has contributed new insights into possible variables and causal mechanisms which may be relevant in the etiology of the disease. Closeness to parents in childhood and the ability to form close interpersonal relationships in later adult life very possibly influence the ability of the individual to cope effectively with environmental stressors prior to neoplastic disease and with the considerable stresses of being a cancer patient subsequent to diagnosis and treatment. Pathogenic pathways for future investigation include mental health variables, such as self-esteem and sense of control at the psychological level and immunity surveillance at the biological. An integration and cross-fertilization of current work in the etiology of and adjustment to cancer is suggested linking psychosomatic and somatopsychic models.

4. Becker, H. **Psychodynamic aspects of breast cancer—differences in younger and older patients.** *Psychother. Psychosom.* 32:287–296, 1979.

We looked into possible differences in the life history and reaction to illness to be observed in younger and older breast cancer patients. The patients, 49 in number, are between 29 and 69 years of age, average age 50. A semi-structured interview took place mostly in the final third of the post-irradiation phase. In the group of women, who developed cancer before the age of 48, some common aspects could be shown in their biography. These women lost an emotionally important person (e.g. a parent) more often in their early childhood. These patients describe an emotionally cold atmosphere in their families along with a missing pronounced basic trust. Also they were overstrained with responsibility too early for their age. The ideals of these patients are somewhat like those of the 'Amazons': they negate the typical female role and its consequences on the bodily, psychic and social level. They seem quite combative, achieving and to the point. As far as sexual responsiveness is concerned only 12% of the younger groups express a consistently positive attitude toward sexuality. Pregnancy, childbirth and breast-feeding are frequently accompanied by serious complications, but they have, in the majority of cases, children. When regarding the multi-causal genesis of cancer, it may be that psychic factors have less influence on the immune system in older patients than the overall ageing process with its weakening of the immunological defence system. The psychic component, if it exists, plays a greater role with the younger patients. The older patients in their life history and pre-morbid behaviour are nearer to what passes for the psychic norm. Other carcinogen factors play a more significant role in older patients: the cancer may have achieved greater autonomy from psychic factors.

5. Bolen, J. S. **Meditation and psychotherapy in the treatment of cancer.** *Psychic.* 4:19–22, 1973.

   ◆ meditation, relaxation, imagery

   Describes the work of an Air Force doctor who combines meditation and cobalt radiation therapy in the treatment of cancer. It is believed that there is a direct correlation between the patient's attitude and his response to cancer therapy. Results of 152 patients treated for cancer show that, for 150 patients, improved or unimproved conditions correlated with their degree of participation and attitudes toward the treatment. 2 patients improved despite negative attitudes. The meditation program, which involves relaxation exercises and visualizations of peaceful scenes, is outlined. The need for experimental validation is discussed.

6. Boranic, M. **The psychophysiological theory of cancer (a review)** (author's transl). *Lijec. Vjesn.* 101:153–158, 1979. (Czechoslovakian)

   The article presents a review of data and theories about the influence of psychogenic factors on the inception and growth of cancer. Patients with cancer are considered to have a personality structure characterized by diminished emotional outlet on the social level. For this reason, regressions of the libidinal energy due to frustrations that have reactivated latent conflicts (e.g. loss of an object), discharge on a more primitive somatic level. By weakening the immunological defence or by disturbing the endocrine function (presumably through the hypothalamus,) this may permit the action of carcinogenic chemicals, viruses and other direct causes of malignant alteration (the "permissive" theory). According to more radical views, the psychic energy might manifest itself on the somatic level as a moving force of an aberrant, persistent cellular growth, the aim of which would be to replace the lost object in a primitive, biological form, so that even the localization of the tumor may serve a symbolic function (the "causative" theory). Cognizance of the psychogenic dimension in the etiology of cancer may find its place in medical measures aimed at prevention and therapy of this disease. For example, preventive actions might be directed toward high-risk individuals who are particularly liable to cancer because of professional, habitual, or personality factors, and the actions might be planned so as to meet their maximal response. On the therapeutic plane, an adequate psychological support to the patients which would promote their general psychophysiological state, might speed up recovery after an operation, irradiation or chemotherapy, and delay or retard the relapses and metastases.

7. Borysenko, J.Z. **Behavioral-physiological factors in the development and management of cancer.** *Gen.Hosp. Psychiatry.* 4:69–74, 1982.

◆ review: relaxation response

Recent clinical and animal model studies have demonstrated an effect of behavioral variables on the course of cancer. Unrelieved anxiety, helplessness, depression, and the inability to modulate the expression of anger have been implicated as specific predictors of poor prognosis. The endocrinological sequelae of these emotional states may affect certain parameters of cell-mediated immunity involved in host resistance to neoplasia. Both corticosteroids and catecholamines are likely mediators of behavioral effects on immunological function. Hormonal variations may also affect growth of tumors directly, or through nonimmunological tissue specific mechanisms. Behavioral interventions based on elicitation of the relaxation response provide a means of influencing affective and physiological states that may have particular relevance to cancer. Practice of such interventions reduces anxiety and provides a substrate for coping that enhances the patient's sense of control. Such "immunization" against helplessness can forestall depression. Physiological effects of such behavioral interventions occur both on a direct and an indirect level. Elicitation of the relaxation response per se produces physiological alterations consistent with decreased arousal of the sympathetic nervous system. Furthermore, by reducing fear and helplessness, physiological changes related to such dysphoric states may be minimized.

8. Cautela, J.R. **Toward a Pavlovian theory of cancer.** *Scand. J. Behav.Ther.* 6:117–142, 1977.

◆ positive reinforcement

Reviews anecdotal and research data indicating that stress and lack of reinforcement (depression, loss) are related to the incidence and growth of cancer. Current theories of the etiology of malignant neoplasma involve cellular abnormalities. Pavlovian theorizing concerning the properties of the nervous system is also focused on cellular functioning. Observations from the Pavlovian laboratories indicate that stress (overstrain of excitatory processes and difficulty in nervous system mobility) and excessive and/or protracted inhibition (lack of reinforcement) produce both behavioral and organic abnormalities. A current view on the etiology of cancer that is being considered seriously is the immunocompetence theory which is consistent with Pavlovian theory on conditioning of the immune system. Preliminary research supports this postulation. Treatment of cancer should involve removal of stress and an increase in the level of reinforcement by behavioral means. The general postulation is that stress and/or lack of reinforcement can provide an environment in which abnormal stimulation can increase the susceptibility to and growth rate of cancer.

9. Chang, J. C. **Nausea and vomiting in cancer patients: an expression of psychological mechanisms?** *Psychosomatics.* 22:707–709, 1981.

◆ placebo, psychotherapy

Extracted summary: Despite the limited effectiveness of cancer therapy, we are now beginning to learn that a patient can be helped a great deal by a careful psychological approach as part of management of the disease. Aside from nausea and vomiting, there are multitudinous complications. Increased attention to psychological aspects may provide us with keener insights into how to help the gravely ill patient cope with the illness. With broader knowledge, we may be able to better manage not only nausea and vomiting, but also the patient's struggle against cancer.

10. Cunningham, A.J. **Psychotherapy for cancer.** *Advances.* 1(4): 8–14, 1984.

    ◆ review: psychotherapy

    Can psychological treatments ameliorate cancer? Alastair J. Cunningham, who recognizes the methodological deficiencies of the clinical studies but who is concerned that their claims may nonetheless be "both true and very important," maintains that another standard should be used to weigh the findings—a standard that might be called the principal of cross-study consistency. Cunningham argues that the results of the clinical studies are consistent with each other and also with the results of prospective studies correlating personality factors with cancer and animal studies investigating the effects of stress on tumor growth. This broad consistency, he suggests, points to a possible core of validity. It indicates, at the very least, that the clinical claims should not be dismissed on methodological grounds and that the time has come to subject the claims to "properly controlled clinical trials."

11. Davis, H.K. **Psychiatry, immunology, and cancer.** *Tex. Med.* 81:49–52, 1985.

    ◆ review: behaviour modification, relaxation, hypnosis, sugestion, imagery, group therapy, biofeedback, doctor-patient relationship, consultation–liaison

    Studies have shown that stress impairs immune system responsiveness and may influence malignant disease. Animal studies, for example, have demonstrated a relationship between stress and accelerated tumor growth, and other studies have suggested a relationship between stress and T and B cell responsiveness. Because of such relationships, physicians treating cancer patients should utilize all available therapies to reduce stress, convey hope, and assure the patient that he or she has allies throughout the illness.

12. Dowling, S.J. **Lourdes cures and their medical assessment.** *J. R. Soc. Med.* 77:634–638, 1984.

◆ spiritual healing

Extracted summary: The latest cure to be passed by the CMIL [International Medical Committee of Lourdes] as medically inexplicable is that of Delizia Cirolli, in September 1982—a child from a village on the slopes of Mount Etna in Sicily. In 1976 when she was 12 years old she presented with a painful swollen right knee. The CMIL studied the case in 1980 and 1981 and at their meeting in 1982 they decided the Ewing's tumour was the correct diagnosis and concluded that the cure was scientifically inexplicable.

13. Feder, S. L. **Psychological considerations in the care of patients with cancer.** *Ann. NY. Acad. Sci.* 125:1020–1027, 1966.

◆ doctor-patient relationship

As physicians, we are concerned with the ultimate outcome of the disease. For the patients, the greatest threat seemed to be not so much that of death, but rather of pain, helplessness, rejection and progressive isolation. Studies of chronically ill people (especially cancer patients who think in terms of disintegration) have shown how intense the fear of abandonment is. It is feared more than death itself. It is usual that we are frightened of things about which we may have some experience or memory. Death is beyond our conscious and unconscious experience (at least subjectively) and cannot be conceptualized; for this reason death is most often equated with abandonment. In the chronically ill person this fear of being unloved and isolated is everywhere. This is what the physician must counteract in every way he can. If our patients are to trust us in this, sympathy and words of reassurance are not enough. If our attitudes and behaviour are determined by our knowledge of the patient's fears and his ways of reacting to them, then we impart a feeling of reassurance he cannot obtain in any other way. Facing the truths with the patient, facing the threat of deterioration, reinforces the trust and the feeling of being wanted. Patients must share their experiences; they are too often not sure they are going to find someone with whom to do it. These have been the immediate humanitarian considerations. There is another issue, perhaps more speculative, but of potential great importance. It is the issue to which this monograph has been directed. This is the hypothesis that psychological factors might play a role not only in the onset of malignant disease, but also in its course. Denial mechanisms are always important in cancer patients. But denial is a poor avenue for emotional discharge. Often it is none at all. The same can be said of the situation where a patient's personal and emotional isolation is increased by the observer's inability to accept the emergent emotions. In avoiding an open relationship and in not offering opportunities for emotional discharge we may be encouraging mechanisms unfavourable to the patient's resistance to the disease. It has been suggested that those patients who have adequate avenues for discharge of tension may have a more favourable later course with cancer than those without such adaptive opportunities. Thus, a greater understanding of the reactions to, and methods of coping with, cancer, some of which have been suggested here, may serve to increase this psycho-physiologic adaptability.

14. Feinstein, A. **Psychological interventions in the treatment of cancer.** *Clin.Psychol. Rev.* 3:1–14, 1983.

◆ review: psychotherapy

Eight variables are identified as being implicated in cancer cases where improvement in disease status has been associated with psychological interventions. Research reports bearing on each of these areas are surveyed, and it is suggested that the variables provide a basis for formulating testable propositions. Clinical research programs could measure changes in medical status following interventions that (1) alter stress conditions and their management, (2) work through unresolved grief, (3) stimulate the will to live, (4) promote realistic positive expectations, (5) mobilize mental capacities for psychophysiological control, (6) constructively handle denial, (7) increase appropriate emotional expression, and (8) strengthen specified personal traits. Considerations related to conducting such research are discussed. Although the nature of any relationship between psychological factors and malignant disease remains unclear, palliative psychological interventions that might also have a beneficial effect on medical status are currently available.

15. Fiore, N. **Fighting cancer—one patient's perspective.** *N.Engl J. Med.* 300:284–289, 1979.

    ◆ psychotherapy, stress management, relaxation, autogenic training, biofeedback, assertiveness training, suggestion, imagery

    Describes the author's experience as a cancer patient (embryonal carcinoma) from diagnosis through the end of chemotherapy. It is emphasized that effective cancer therapy must treat the healthy portions of the patient's body and psyche as well as the diseased cells. Suggestions for using individual psychotherapy sessions at different points in cancer therapy are presented.

16. Forester, B., Kornfeld, D. S. and Fleiss, J. L. **Psychotherapy during radiotherapy: effects on emotional and physical distress.** *Am. J. Psychiatry.* 142:22–27, 1985.

    ◆ psychotherapy

    The authors determined the effects of ongoing weekly individual psychotherapy on the symptoms of patients undergoing a 6-week course of radiotherapy for cancer. Forty-eight patients were given weekly psychotherapy sessions for 10 weeks; another 52 patients served as control subjects. A statistically significant reduction was found in both emotional and "physical" manifestations of distress in the patients receiving psychotherapy compared with the control group. This was true regardless of gender, ward or private patient status, or knowledge of diagnosis. Patient gender and knowledge of diagnosis did affect the pattern and magnitude of the response to psychotherapy.

17. Greer, S. Morris, T. and Pettingale, K. W. **Psychological response to breast cancer: effect on outcome.** *Lancet.* 2:785–787, 1979.

A prospective, multidisciplinary, 5-year study of 69 consecutive female patients with early ($T_{0,1}$ $N_{0,1}$ M_0) breast cancer was conducted. Patients' psychological responses to the diagnosis of cancer was assessed 3 months postoperatively. These responses were related to outcome 5 years after operation. Recurrence-free survival was significantly common among patients who had initially reacted to cancer by denial or who had a fighting spirit than among patients who had responded with stoic acceptance or feelings of helplessness and hopelessness.

18. Greer, S. and Morris, T. **The study of psychological factors in breast cancer: problems of method.** *Soc. Sci. Med.* 12:129–134, 1978.

160 women admitted consecutively for breast tumor biopsy were interviewed and assessed on the Hamilton Rating Scale for Depression, the Eysenck Personality Inventory, and the Hostility-Direction of Hostility Questionnaire. At operation, 69 subjects were diagnosed as having breast cancer (BC) and 91 as having benign breast disease; the latter group served as controls. A major result of statistical comparisons was a significant correlation between the diagnosis of BC and a behavioral pattern, persisting throughout adult life, of abnormal release of anger. This abnormality was, in most cases, extreme suppression. Although major sources of bias were avoided in the present study, critical examination of its methods shows several limitations. It is suggested that further advances in this area depend on more stringent methods, and several recommendations are presented concerning such methods.

19. Le Shan, L. L., Gassmann, M. L. **Some observations on psychotherapy with patients suffering from neoplastic disease.** *Am. J. Psychother.* 12:733–734, 1958.

◆ psychotherapy

Ten patients with malignant neoplasms were studied in over 1400 hours of intensive depth psychotherapy. This led to the recognition of a number of special problems arising during the psychotherapeutic treatment of cancer patients. Some tentative methods of handling these problems are presented and it is hoped that they will prove useful to others working in the same field. The special problems were divided into four areas: (1) the anxieties of the cancer patient. These are predominantly realistic in nature and have to be accepted as such. More support is needed in this form of treatment than is generally given during psychotherapy. (2) The anxieties of the therapist. The therapist must be clear about the goals and values of working with patients who are likely to die in the course of the process. A control therapist is necessary in order that the stress, when one patient dies, does not affect the therapist's relationships with the other cancer patients. (3) The personality of cancer patients. Certain personality factors which have implications for therapy appear with a good deal of consistency in individuals with cancer. These include an unusual amount of deeply repressed hostility, marked feelings of psychological isolation, and despair about having been unable to achieve real satisfactions in life. (4) Special psychosomatic aspects. There is some reason to believe that psychotherapy may under certain circumstances affect the growth rate and development of neoplasms. Therefore a good deal of caution is recommended in deciding how much guilt and hostility may be mobilized during the therapeutic process.

20. Levy, S. M. **Emotions and the progression of cancer: a review.** *Advances*. 1:10–15, 1984.

◆ review: doctor-patient relationship, relaxation, imagery

Extracted summary: If the argument to this point is correct—that lower survival rates from cancer are associated with depression or helplessness and higher rates are associated with a sense of coping—then the question must be asked: can helplessness and the lack of coping among cancer patients be altered? And if they can, will the change affect the outcome of the disease? The answer to the first question is undoubtedly yes. The strategies for change are numerous. In some, the patient's outlook is the target. The literature indicates that various cognitive interventions—for example, role rehearsal, self-rewards, and thought stoppage—alter depressive or helpless behaviour. A recent article by Peterson suggests that medical practitioners adapt for use with patients the type of strategies that dispel helplessness in animals. Peterson suggests that a physician could enlist patients as collaborators in their own treatment, explaining to them that their progress depended on this assistance. Patients thus would be led ......(page 227 missing)

21. Meares, A. **Regression of recurrence of carcinoma of the breast at mastectomy site associated with intensive meditation.** *Aust. Fam. Physician.* 10:218–219, 1981.

    ◆ meditation

    Extracted summary: The patient attended each weekday for a month of intensive meditation. By this time there was clear evidence of healing. It was arranged that the patient should return to her home in another State, and come back for further treatment in a month's time. However, by then the ulcer had nearly healed, the patient said she was well and felt it was unnecessary to return for further treatment. Figure 2 shows the ulcer completely healed, and the hard raised nodules have disappeared. She has however, recently developed a bony metastasis for which she has had cobalt radiation.

22. Meares, A. **What can the cancer patient expect from intensive meditation?** *Aust. Fam. Physician,* 9:322–325, 1980.

    ◆ meditation

    The results of treatment of 73 patients with advanced cancer who have been able to attend at least 20 sessions of intensive meditation, indicates that nearly all such patients should expect significant reduction of anxiety and depression, together with much less discomfort and pain. There is reason to expect a ten per cent chance of quite remarkable slowing of the rate of growth of the tumour, and a ten per cent chance of less marked but still significant slowing. The results indicate that patients with advanced cancer have a ten per cent chance of regression of the growth. There is a fifty per cent chance of greatly improved quality of life and for those who die, a ninety per cent chance of death with dignity.

23. Nieburgs, H. E., Weiss, J., Navarrete, M., Strax, P., Teirstein, A., Grillione, G., and Siedlecki, B. **The role of stress in human and experimental oncogenesis.** *Cancer Detect. Prev.* 2:307–36, 1979.

A series of experiments were carried out to determine the effects of stress at the cellular level. This report is based upon the action of electric shock, forced cold swim, and handling on cellular changes in the gastric mucosa, liver, thymus, adrenals and blood lymphocytes. Two hour electric shock was associated with increased secretory granules in gastric chief cells, liver mitoses and marked lymphopenia. Use of 24-hour shock revealed less secretory granules, absence of liver mitoses, and only slight lymphopenia with delayed but longer lasting effects. Stress consistently produced a marked decrease in the number of small lymphocytes, with an increase in medium-sized lymphocytes and usually also in large lymphocytes, the latter depending upon the kind of stressor and the length of period following cessation of stress. Changes in the proportion of lymphocytes, particularly the decreased percentage of small lymphocytes, was closely related to the increase in liver mitoses. Control animals also revealed blood lymphocyte changes following repeated removal of rats from the same environment. Stress-induced effects from transportation of rats were evident by changes in gastric chief cells and liver mitoses for 12 to 16 days after shipment. Stress by electric shock immediately after transportation produced less effects than shock applied at least 21 days following animal transportation. Comparison of effects from various stressors revealed that lymphocyte changes persisted for 72 hours following handling and cold swim. Whereas liver mitoses were present in all rats at 96 hours, thymus involution was noted at 72 hours following handling, 48 hours after cold swim and 96 hours after electric shock. Slight adrenal hypertrophy persisted for 96 hours following handling and shock and for 24 hours after cold swim. The effect of stress on DMBA mammary tumorigenesis differed in relation to the kind of stressor and the length of the stress period following DMBA administration. At 90 days, cold swim and handling enhanced tumor induction, whereas, electric shock inhibited tumor induction but enhanced the rate of tumor growth. At 150 days, the number of rats with tumors was slightly greater and the tumor size considerably smaller in stressed rats than in those without stress following DMBA administration. The inhibited tumor growth of DMBA treated rats that were stressed for 150 days by handling and cold swim was associated with an increase in large- and medium-sized lymphocytes, and a marked decrease in small lymphocytes. The same increase in large- and medium-sized lymphocytes, and the marked decrease in small lymphocytes, also occurred in women with repressed hostility and in patients with a family history of cancer, as well as in patients with breast cancer and with poorly differentiated and metastatic lung cancer. The close relationship between a decrease in small lymphocytes and increase in identifiable liver mitoses points to a regulatory function of small lymphocytes (T lymphocytes) on cell kinetics. Possibly the entire imbalance of decreased small lymphocytes with markedly increased medium-sized and large lymphocytes may be responsible for the prolonged mitotic phases as evidenced from presence of mitoses. The imbalance in the proportion of lymphocytes as a result of stress, and the consistently found decrease of small lymphocytes with an increase in medium sized and large lymphocytes in cancer patients suggests a possible role of stress in the multifactorial etiology of neoplastic disease.

24. Peter, B. and Gerl, W. **Hypnotherapy in the psychologic treatment of cancer.** *Hypn. Kognition*. 1:56–68, 1984. (in German)

◆ psychotherapy, hypnosis

A report of the author's psychotherapeutic and hypnotherapeutic work with cancer patients. Among the topics discussed are hypnotherapy for the control of pain and other side effects of the disease and its treatment, hypnotherapeutic activation of the body's immune system and unconscious coping mechanism, hypnotherapeutic stimulation of the will to live, and hypnotherapy as a means to support the patient in coping with the illness.

25. Redd, W. H. and Andrykowski, M. A. **Behavioral intervention in cancer treatment: controlling aversion reactions to chemotherapy.** *J. Consult. Clin. Psychol.* 50:1018–1029. 1982.

◆ hypnosis, imagery, relaxation, desensitization

During the protracted course of cancer chemotherapy, approximately 25% of patients develop aversion reactions to treatment by becoming nauseated and/or vomiting before their chemotherapy treatments. This phenomenon has been conceptualized as a result of respondent conditioning. Since commonly used antiemetic drugs do not reliably control anticipatory nausea/emesis, behavioral techniques of control have been studied. They include hypnosis used in conjunction with guided-relaxation imagery, progressive muscle relaxation with guided imagery, and systematic desensitization.

26. Redd, W. H. and Hendler-Cobie, S. **Behavioral medicine in comprehensive cancer treatment.** *J. Psychosoc. Oncol.* 1:3–17, 1983.

◆ behaviour therapy

The application of principles of behavioral psychology to treat aversion reactions to chemotherapy, fear of medical procedures, and psychosomatic symptoms in adult and pediatric cancer patients represents a broadening of psychosocial oncology's domain. The authors discuss these applications, focusing on theoretical premises of behavioral medicine and on specific clinical examples. Attention is also given to the integration of behavioral medicine within comprehensive cancer treatment. It is argued that this new area of psychosocial oncology provides an effective means of treating previously unaddressed problems and is compatible with other approaches.

27. Redd, W. H. and Hendler-Cobie, S. **Learned aversions to chemotherapy treatment.** *Health Educ. Q.* 10:57–66, 1984.

◆ hypnosis, imagery, relaxation, biofeedback, desensitization

Recent advances in behavioral psychology and its application in medical settings have yielded effective methods for reducing distress in patients undergoing cancer treatment. The present authors discuss the control of anticipatory nausea and vomiting in patients receiving chemotherapy. The development of these symptoms is hypothesized to be of psychopathological or physiological origin, or due to respondent conditioning. Antiemetic drugs are generally unreliable in their control of chemotherapy nausea, especially with conditioned aversions, and may produce side effects of their own. Four behavioral methods—hypnosis used with guided imagery, progressive muscle relaxation training with imagery, biofeedback with imagery, and systematic desensitization—and their uses and results are described. Clinically significant reductions in patient reactions were achieved despite large variations in the type of cancer, stage of the disease, and chemotherapy protocol. The applications of behavioral interventions to other types of cancer treatments are discussed.

28. Renneker, R. E., Cutler, R., Hora, J., Bradley, G., Kearney, J. and Cutler, M. **Psychoanalytical explorations of emotional correlates of cancer of the breast.** *Psychosom. Med.* 25:106–123, 1963.

    ◆ psychotherapy

    Extracted summary: It is our belief that psychotherapy is indicated in all major or life-threatening organic conditions which grow out of the soil of a depression. Treatment should be vigorous, active, and directed primarily against the dynamics of the depression. Psychotherapy is also indicated in a patient with cancer of the breast when psychiatric evaluation discloses a neurotic system decompensating in the areas and ways described in this report. Treatment aims at the replacement of object-fixated, frustrated drives with sublimatory outlets or new relatively conflict-free objects. If psychotherapy contributed to the longevity of any patient, then it possibly accomplished this by raising host resistance through achievement of these aims.

29. Rowden, L. **Relaxation and visualisation techniques in patients with breast cancer.** *Nurs. Times.* 80:42–44, 1984.

    ◆ review: relaxation, imagery

    Extracted summary: On a personal note, I have found that

relaxation has helped me deal with daunting situations with some success. This is obviously a subjective opinion, as are those held by the patients I meet who use the techniques and feel helped. I recognize the difficulty of assessing such techniques because of the different methods which can be used and the sceptical views of many of our colleagues. The growing demand for a holistic approach to care requires a research programme to evaluate scientifically these previously untested modes of therapy for the cancer patient.

30. Schonfield, J. **Psychological factors related to recovery from breast cancer** (abstract). *Psychosom. Med.* 39:51, 1977.

Do psychological factors play any role in the recurrence of early carcinomas of the breast? Forty nine women with Stage I, II or III breast cancer, who had previously undergone either a partial or radical mastectomy, were interviewed during the first week of radiation therapy. They were also asked to answer 128 items from the MMPI and a forty item disguised measure of anxiety. Two years after radiotherapy the medical status of all 49 women was obtained, and two groups were formed: (1) a group with no evidence of recurrence at that time (N=37), and (2) a group with clear evidence of recurrence who were either still alive or who had died from their disease within two years (N=12). No relationship was found between the initial stage of the disease and recurrence or non-recurrence. The group with no recurrence had significantly higher scores on an MMPI scale measuring physical well-being and significantly lower scores on the hypochondriasis scale of the MMPI. The group with a recurrence had significantly higher scores on the frustrative tension sub-scale of the anxiety measure. Just short of statistical significance ($p<10$) was the score on the Morale Loss (severe depression) scale of the MMPI, where the group with a recurrence scored higher than the group without. The overall picture that emerges is that the women who survived two years post breast surgery and radiotherapy without any recurrence were less anxious initially and were possibly also less depressed. All the scales with significant results in the present study (with the exception of the hypocondriasis scale) have also been found to differentiate in the same direction, cancer patients undergoing radiotherapy who do, or do not return to gainful employment one year later, when all were in remission status. It would appear that these personality scales are tapping characteristics important both to the adjustment to having had cancer, and in the length of survival from this disease.

31. Shapiro, A. **Psychotherapy as adjunct treatment for cancer patients.** *Am. J. Clin. Hypn.* 25:150–155, 1982.

    ◆ psychotherapy, hypnosis, imagery

    Describes the progress of 2 cancer patients in psychotherapy who used the ability to minimize pain and discomfort, maintain a high white cell count despite ongoing chemotherapy, and augment the ability of the body's immune system to fight the disease. All were accomplished through the use of visual imagery in the trance state. Visual imagery was also used to reach feelings that subjects were often unable to verbalize. The gradual shift from despair to hope and even confidence, as well as the development of more assertive behavior, is discussed.

32. Shekelle, R. B., Raynor, W. J., Ostfeld, A. M., Garron, D. C., Bieliauskas, L., Liu, S. C., Maliza, C. and Paul, O. **Psychological depression and 17-year risk of death from cancer.** *Psychosom. Med.* 43:117–125, 1981.

    Psychological depression; measured in 1957–1958 by the Minnesota Multiphasic Personality Inventory at the baseline examination of 2,020 middle-aged employed men, was associated ($p<0.001$) with a twofold increase in odds of death from cancer during 17 years of follow-up. The association did not vary appreciably in magnitude among the early (1958–1962), middle (1963–1968), and later (1969–1974) years of follow-up, persisted after adjustment for age, cigarette smoking, use of alcohol, family history of cancer, and occupational status, and was apparently not specific to any particular site or type of cancer. This result, predicted in advance on the basis of findings by other investigators, is consistent with the hypothesis that psychological depression is related to impairment of mechanisms for preventing the establishment and spread of

33. Simonton, O. C., Matthews-Simonton, S. and Sparks, T. F. **Psychological intervention in the treatment of cancer.** *Psychosomatics*. 21:226–233, 1980.

◆ psychotherapy

In a preliminary study of the effects of psychological intervention in the treatment of advanced cancer, it was found that patients so treated survived up to twice as long as would have been expected based on national averages. Better patient motivation, greater confidence in the treatment, and overall positive expectancy are thought to have contributed to the results. An educational model has been developed employing the psychological processes used in the study, and further investigations are under way to assess the effect of the patient's mental health on the course of cancer.

34. Spiegel, Bernie., M.D. **Love, Medicine and Miracles** (Published by Harper Perennial.

35. Stenlin, J. S. Jr. and Brach, K. H. **Psychological aspects of cancer therapy: a surgeon's viewpoint.** *JAMA*.. 197:100–104, 1966.

◆ doctor-patient relationship

With regard to his attitude toward cancer, the patient (and the physician as well) consciously or unconsciously equates the word "cancer" with death—death in its worst form, perhaps next month, next week, or even tomorrow. Frequently, his attitude is based upon erroneous information concerning a friend who had cancer, or upon a distressing recollection of a relative who died of the disease. Open discussion of this problem can go far toward reassuring the patient and allaying his fears. Since most malignant processes apparently develop slowly, the patient should be given to understand that his cancer did not begin yesterday; rather, he has probably been living with it for months or years, and still more important, he will not be dead tomorrow. He should also be made to understand that all cancers are not alike and that many patients with certain forms of the disease, although incurable, have lived productive lives for long periods of time, just as they have lived with chronic nonmalignant processes. Here, the surgeon can suggest that the patient's natural body resistance may be effective in controlling the disease. It is well established that an occasional patient with cancer has a resistance to its spread. Is it not possible that this particular patient may be one of these fortunate ones? The physical aspects of the patient's cancer and the therapeutic measures available obviously influence the quality of hope he may be offered. At this stage, the surgeon's approach must be directed toward hope for control of the cancer, rather than hope for the cure. First, the surgeon is well justified in pointing out the possibility of control of the cancer by the clinical measures available for this purpose. Aggressive surgical procedures, well-planned radiotherapy, hormones, steroids, and other forms of chemotherapy have proved valuable adjuncts to the supportive care of these patients. The senior author makes no apology for administering chemotherapeutic drugs in moderate doses and under well-controlled circumstances, even to patients with cancers that are known to respond poorly. Their usage in this manner is justified, if for no other reason than to show the patient that a positive attempt is being made to retard the progress of the disease. The physician who refuses to adopt an attitude to hopelessness and despair toward patients with advanced cancer may succeed in adding worthwhile years to the lives of some of those otherwise doomed to early and miserable death, and on rare occasions may bring about cure.

36. Weinstock, C. **Recent progress in cancer psychobiology and psychiatry.** *J. Am. Soc. Psychosom. Dent. Med.* 24:4–14, 1977.

◆ psychotherapy

A specific pattern preceding the onset of cancer has been identified in many patients: extensive trauma experienced in the 1st 7 years of life, impaired trust in parents, and fostered repression of anger. These patients were generally unable to form strong attachments, and one satisfying object relationship occurring in young adulthood was later lost, resulting in hopeless depression. Cancer followed within 6 mo to 8 yrs. Location of the tumor may follow symbolic principles; e.g. in the brain in unfulfilled intellectuals, and in the sex organs in homosexuals. Amelioration of the depression—whether through improved family relations, etc., or psychotherapy—

precedes many cases of so-called spontaneous regression of the cancer. Psychotherapy should focus upon mobilization of grief and the search for a new object in life.

37. Weitz, R. D. **Psychological factors in the prevention and treatment of cancer.** *Psychother. Private Pract.* 1:69–76, 1983.

◆ hypnosis, imagery

Discusses mind and body interaction relative to the development of disease process, particularly cancer. The role of stress as a significant factor in the breakdown of the body's immune system is analyzed. The author's experience with the use of hypnosis and imagery as ancillary therapeutic interventions is described and evaluated. It is noted that personality variables are observed in previous research with cancer patients: many cancer patients have experienced a significant emotional trauma 6–18 mo before cancer is evidenced. It is concluded that individuals have potential in exerting control over their lives and producing a lifestyle that is relatively free of the forces leading to illness. The psychologist has a significant role to play in this emphasis on health maintenance. A national communication network is recommended to consolidate the observations of psychological clinicians working with cancer.

APPENDIX III
HOW CAN AUSTRALIAN WOMEN DIAGNOSED WITH BREAST CANCER BE HELPED BEST?

Dr. Ian Gawler OAM, BVSc
The Gawler Foundation

PRELIMINARY REMARKS

A diagnosis of breast cancer is usually shattering—a great shock for most women. With their lives and family in crisis, they are often then required to make rapid decisions concerning treatment and subsequent life changes. The treatment generally involves surgery which frequently includes removal of a breast and usually challenges the woman's body image and sexuality dramatically. Subsequent chemotherapy and/or radiotherapy can be physically debilitating and psychologically demanding.

It is not surprising that women in this situation often are shocked, depressed, confused, traumatised. This reaction is not unique to women with breast cancer, it is a common initial response to a diagnosis of cancer by men or women. Women's ability to suffer nobly in these circumstances and to rise above that suffering is often extraordinary. For example, see the extraordinary case history of Joyce Oag, **Appendix A**. Yet the acceptance by the women themselves, and the community generally, that this suffering is acceptable, may well be in part a sexist issue and certainly is not acceptable.

To alleviate their suffering, there is an urgent need to provide compassionate, high quality care at every level for women diagnosed with breast cancer. This cannot be said to be happening at the moment, although powerful signs of improvement are appearing.

The Gawler Foundation—representing the patient's perspective

The Gawler Foundation is perhaps Australia's best known and well respected patient and community based, self-help organisation which has a particular focus on helping people affected by cancer.

The Foundation's submission aims to examine the issues and provide answers that could improve breast cancer management—from the perspective of the patients and families concerned. No doubt many other submissions will examine the proposition from the outside—from the perspective of the medical profession or other helping, caring bodies. Having conducted support groups since 1981 and having around 10,000 people attend these groups, this submission aims to represent the patients and present their point of view.

Three Major Observations

1. Each "case" to be treated as an individual

While statistics and generalisations are useful, there needs to be a basic observation made. Every individual woman's experience of breast cancer is intensely personal and unique. Effective management of breast cancer will require a flexible system with a coordinated staff and range of resources that can assess, respond to and satisfy the reactions and needs of each individual woman.

2. The need for a paradigm shift in research and treatment

The Foundation contends that a radical shift in the paradigm of cancer treatment is required. Radical surgery, most chemotherapies and radiotherapy may be the best treatments of our day. However, while they remain so devastating in their effects upon the patients, they can never be fully satisfactory, and therefore, acceptable. While a woman may be relatively happy to survive breast cancer following a mastectomy, obviously it would seem better to survive with her breast intact.

This proposition—to search for non toxic, non invasive solutions to cancer seems to provoke major and often emotional reactions from the cancer authorities of today. It is unfortunate that some alternative cancer cures have used emotional rhetoric and unscientific methods to promote these aims. The Gawler Foundation is not interested in that approach. We are talking of the humane treatment of fragile human beings at a time of great distress and vulnerability. We do not represent an "alternative" view; but are vitally concerned to combine all the best resources to help the people involved best.

It is clear that new areas of research must be followed, new solutions sought and found. The fact is that a woman's chances of surviving breast cancer are only slightly better today than they were 20 years ago—despite billions of dollars of research all around the world.

Professor Lowenthal says that "taken overall, science has made only a modest impact on the problem of cancer ... Even where effective treatments can be offered, to many patients the potential side effects of surgery, radiotherapy and chemotherapy are perceived as unacceptable relative to their possible benefits."

It is hard to image this volume of unproductive research receiving ongoing support in any other business than the cancer industry.

The Foundation contends that the approach to cancer research and treatment needs to change. Even if a new heavy chemotherapy was found to be 100% effective, we contend it would still be essentially unsatisfactory as it is too hard on the patient.

Research should continue urgently with a focus on finding a more "patient-friendly" cure. The indication presently is that such answers are likely to be found in the realm of the immune system and the mind and spirit of the patient.

3. Support Groups and Mind/Body Medicine

In 1989, Spiegel, in his now famous study, reported in *The Lancet* that women with secondary breast cancer doubled their survival times by attending a support group. Spiegel's study focuses a great deal of other research that indicates people can clearly help themselves and that self help techniques can offer major gains in quality of life and survival times.

If Spiegel's wonderful results had been due to a new drug, we contend it would be advocated for virtually every new patient by now. Yet a common complaint of members of our groups is that they were not told by medical staff of self help options and their possibility. And while many members are recommended to our self help programs by their doctors and have their active support, many still complain that their doctors oppose their attendance.

The "anecdotal" evidence provided by the lives and stories of thousands of people who have attended support groups is overwhelming. The creditable scientific research also is massive. (See **Appendix B for** a Major review of this presented in the *Australian Doctor*, 1993).

Cancer Support Groups deserve immediate and ongoing support on all levels. Active cancer support groups have proven their worth. They are well established, if still at a fledgling stage. They provide an essential service that has been proven to enhance quality of life and improve survival times of women with breast cancer. They deserve support through encouragement and funding.

A summary of recommendations appears at the end of our written submission.

SUBMISSION FROM THE GAWLER FOUNDATION

The Basic Facts of Breast Cancer are Well Known

- A woman's risk of developing breast cancer in her life time is, depending on her country, 1 in 12 to 1 in 15.
- Only approximately 50% of women diagnosed with breast cancer are alive 5 years later.
- If breast cancer has spread into the nearby skin or muscle or spread to the nodes in the neck, medically there is only a tiny chance of complete or permanent cure.
- Early detection does improve survival chances.
- There is a powerful correlation between fat consumption and incidence of breast cancer.
- Attending a cancer support group has been shown to dramatically improve quality of life, and double survival times.

A more extensive overview of breast cancer is presented in The Gawler Foundation's fact sheet on the topic—see **Appendix C.**

Women turn to the Medical Profession for Primary Treatment—but many problems are reported.

In 1991, Dr. Gawler was invited to present a paper to the RACGP conference. At this Conference research was presented that had been gathered from around 100 cancer patients and partners who attended Foundation programs. The patients were not all breast cancer patients but the results are presented as typical.

The questions researched were:

1. Where is the medical system being effective in cancer management?
2. Where is the system ineffective?
3. What could doctors do to help you better?

A full summary is presented as **Appendix D.**

The most important points can be summarised as:

1. Patients turn to the medical profession for primary care but are often disappointed.
2. The disappointment is usually more to do with communication and interpersonal skills than technical or treatment issues.
3. Patients are seeking better levels of communication and more enthusiasm and support for Self Help techniques.
4. Patients are seeking doctors they can work with as partners in a cooperative, healing endeavour.

Decisions Regarding Treatment Pose Special Difficulties

A study in the New Scientist in 1986 examined treatments recommended by different doctors for the treatment of two imaginary patients. For a sample patient with a poor prognosis, 62 doctors suggested 36 different plans of treatment. For the patient with a good prognosis, 53 doctors recommended 42 different plants. Compared with their Scottish counterparts, Australian doctors were far more likely to recommend an extended mastectomy and to prescribe chemotherapy for both types of patients.

In plain English, this means that if a woman with breast cancer with a good prognosis went to another doctor for a confirming second opinion, she could consult 43 doctors before she found it!

The situation is little better today as the article "Doubts on breast treatment" *Australian Doctor* (18th february 1994) demonstrate—see **Appendix E.**

A woman with extensive breast cancer, will have a 2 in 3 chance of gaining a remission with combination chemotherapy but even so her average life expectancy is only 21 months.

In at least 80% of breast cancers, removal of the lump only, not the whole breast, is adequate and for many women, preferable. Yet many women are still recommended full mastectomies.

This all points to the difficulty of the choices to consider and the need for compassionate, professional advice backed by excellent communication skills.

Active Cancer Support Groups offer the Opportunity to talk, be listened to and to learn self help techniques.

Clearly women in Australia diagnosed with breast cancer need better support than they have been receiving through mainstream channels. Clearly too, active cancer support groups can meet the need of support. They will have the added bonus of teaching life skills that can translate into improved quality of life and longer survival times.

What is meant by an Active Cancer Support Group?

Cancer support groups can be classified in 3 ways:

(i) Passive support groups: While these groups do pay attention to patient needs, they seem to be concerned primarily with facilitating the medical management of the disease. These groups help explain the nature of medical treatments, assist with transport needs, provide cups of tea, reassurance and a chance to talk with others. They are often run by medical staff and seem fairly to be described as medically based, treatment support groups. The emphasis is on helping patients to attend and comply with treatments, and improving quality of life. The notion of improving survival times by attending is usually frowned upon by these groups.

(ii) Discussion based Cancer Support Groups: These groups usually provide a safe and skilled forum in which members can discuss their problems and share experiences. Teaching a range of self help techniques is not a part of these groups charter and is often positively avoided; although relaxation and/or meditation is often a part of the sessions—as in Spiegel's groups. Usually they emphasise the quality of life benefits. For example, Spiegel told women joining his groups that he did not expect any improvement in survival times as a result of attending the groups. He was quite surprised himself by the outcome. Apparently the improved quality of life, the relaxation and meditation, the mutual support and other benefits of the group did translate directly into longer survival.

(iii) Active Cancer Support Groups: These have the stated intentions of providing mutual support and teaching life skills. The emphasis is dual—to improve quality of life and improve survival times—through the teaching of self help techniques.

In earlier days, the whole area of self help techniques seems to have been very challenging to the medical cancer specialists and hierarchy. For a long time it seems that oncologists have held the view that the only way a patient with cancer can get better is if they respond to medical treatment.

Cancer patients have been singled out as apparently being particularly vulnerable and weak headed. There is a special section in the Victorian State Medical Practitioners Act Section 28(8) which says that,

> "Any unregistered person who directly or indirectly demands or receives any fee or reward whatsoever for or in connection with treatment or advice in relation to cancer or any disease or condition which he alleges to be cancer shall be guilty of an offence against this Act unless in the case of each person treated or advised the giving of such treatment or advice is expressly authorised by a legally qualified medical practitioner.
>
> Penalty:
>
> For a first offence—10 penalty units.
>
> For a second or subsequent offence—20 penalty units or imprisonment for two years".

To apply this section in its strictest interpretation would be a nonsense. It means that to advise a friend with cancer to lie down and have a cup of tea, would be to break the law.

However, its interpretation certainly clouds what a support group can do legally; it certainly clouds what non-medical health practitioners (such as natural therapists) can do. This, of course, clouds patients' freedom to choose how they might like to manage their own illness. This section of the Victorian Act needs revision.

How the Gawler Foundation Supports Women with Breast Cancer

The Gawler Foundation's cancer support is based around four main programs. (Summary of all Foundation services, **Appendix F**).

(i) **The 12 week cancer support group.** This program has been running continuously since 1981 and around 6000 people have attended it. The program has used the same format since 1981 while the content has evolved based on patient feedback and new insights and research. The emphasis is on learning self help techniques, especially eating well, developing a positive state of mind, meditation and mutual support. Program Details—**Appendix G.**

In 1993, only 7 women with breast cancer attended this program. Their ages ranged from 28 to 60 years. Two attended with partners. All were from Victoria (local area).

(ii) **The ongoing cancer support group.** Designed to meet the needs of ongoing support after the initial 12 weeks, these groups have strong elements of the discussion type support groups, while reinforcing and problem solving self help techniques.

(iii) **The 10 day residential program.** Running at around one program per month since 1985, this live-in program makes attendance easier for distant patients, while providing a more concentrated introduction to this approach. Around 4000 have attended this program.

In 1993, 337 people attended this program. Of those 55 were women with breast cancer. They ranged in age from 34 to 66; the average age was 46. 23 came from Victoria, 14 from NSW, 8 from Queensland, 2 from NT, 0 from SA, 1 from WA, 1 from Tasmania, 4 from New Zealand, one from UK and one from Denmark. Of the 55 only 19 came with partners. This represents 29%, whereas for the whole year an average of 47% of all patients attended with partners. Our feeling is that a significant number of women with breast cancer lack good support, even when it comes to their partners. In this situation an active support group helps fill a very real need, very effectively. The Residential program is presented in **Appendix H.**

(iv) **The 5 day Follow Up Residential Program**. Usually run every six months, this program provides further learning time, problem solving and more time out for members to focus on their own needs.

These programs are supported by access to counselling via telephone and in person, special conferences and workshops, books, tapes and other resources. The Foundation makes an ongoing commitment to provide follow up support. A summary of all the Foundation Services is presented as **Appendix F.**

What are the benefits of attending a Cancer Support Group?

Answer: Improvements in Quality of Life and Survival Times!

Most of our patients, particularly women with breast cancer, believe that stress helped to precipitate their cancer. Certainly the diagnosis commonly creates major stress. There is overwhelming evidence to demonstrate that negative stress weakens the immune system and that this can predispose the body to developing cancer and/or weaken its chance of recovery. A lengthy list of Medical References covering this and other aspects of the Foundation's work is included in **Appendix I.**

Happily it is also being demonstrated that a positive state of mind backed by good nutrition can enhance immune function and has the powerful possibility of increasing survival times. In simple terms hope, faith, love and joy while obviously constituting the elements of a good quality of life, do translate into improved survival times. Common sense always said that this was so. Modern science, particularly psycho-neuroimmunology (or mind/body medicine) is establishing why and how this is so.

In the past patients basically were left to cope on their own. If they "happened" to have a positive nature, they generally "happened" to do better than those with a negative disposition.

Happily, an active cancer support group can provide positive intervention and teach a negative person how to become more positive. This is achieved through a variety of strategies, many of which are a unique function of the group itself. In the words of Dr. Robert Proctor (a Melbourne psychiatrist who ran sessions for The Foundation's 12 week program for several years):

> "An effective way to help such people come to this awareness is via an intensive group experience such as has been initiated by Ian Gawler. The group experience is far more powerful than one-on-one therapy, as people

gain great value from the shared accounts of other patients' insights and experiences and the great sense of support and camaraderie that develops in such a healing and learning environment.

I strongly recommend that all cancer patients be offered the opportunity to participate in such a group process, either as an "in-house" program at their treating hospital or at some external centre."

What Financial Benefits may there be to the Government?

We contend that women attending a cancer support group are likely to become more independent and self reliant. There is good grounds to believe that this would translate directly into less dependence on Institutional care and so save the Health System significant resources and money. This is an area warranting major research which the Foundation is keen to participate in.

What are the necessary conditions for a successful Active Cancer Support Group?

1. It should be seen to be patient based and focused on meeting the needs of patients, families and friends.

One of the Gawler Foundation's strengths is our independence and integrity. We have no affiliation to individuals, groups or bodies that compromise our commitment to serving those affected by cancer. We have no commitment to any particular method, other than finding what might best help a given individual. This is clear to all who attend and so generates trust and confidence in what we offer.

2. It should be based on the experiences and knowledge of other, successful patients and their supporters. The Foundation began with Ian and Grace Gawler sharing what had worked for them during Ian's recovery from osteogenic sarcoma. That initial experience has been added to by the feedback gained from over 10,000 members of our groups. This means that the Foundation acts as a pool of patient based experience. We are able to discuss what has worked for others and what has not. Most people attending Foundation programs are in the above

> average socio-economic range. Most make many enquiries, read many books and can fairly be described as "expert" patients! Their pool of knowledge and experience is invaluable and forms the basis of what our programs offer to new members.

What is the attitude to Doctors really like?

Again their seems to be a stumbling block in some quarters that groups like ours are anti-medical. This is not so. It is fair to say that as patient advocates we probably should be more active in pointing out the deficiencies in the existing medical system—and the successes. As already stated, there are major concerns with levels of communication between Doctors and their patients, and with the personal cost of many treatments.

However our support groups often have the effect of helping patients to overcome what are often very natural fears and reservations, and to return for effective medical treatments.

It has to be said that women with advanced secondary breast cancer have very difficult decisions to make regarding treatment. In some instances quality of life considerations may suggest no treatment is in the patient's best interests. There is a problem that not all doctors take a balanced view in these matters. We do encourage patients and families to assert their rights, to ask questions, demand answers and assume responsibility for their own decisions if that is what they want to do. We also support their right to allow a doctor to make those hard decisions for them—if that is the patient's choice.

Overall, let us state again: we are committed to supporting patients. The vast majority of patients want the best medical care available backed by the best self help techniques they can learn and practise.

Training—sharing the knowledge and experience

The Gawler Foundation has offered training for leaders of like-minded, active cancer support groups since 1988. Groups in each capital City have been helped to develop and each runs as an autonomous body. Most are incorporated Associations in their States, as the Gawler Foundation is in Victoria.

While some groups are running in country areas, we believe that there is an urgent need to help more begin and continue.

Importantly, suitability for leading these types of cancer support groups is often better determined by life experience, particularly that with cancer, than academic qualifications.

For the Future

There is an immediate need for a National Body to coordinate, train and regulate active cancer support groups. Like most Professional Bodies, this will best be achieved by peers and should remain in the domain of the patients and supporters themselves.

The Foundation is committed to maintaining an active role in training and supporting other groups and would be happy to liaise or act as consultants to new initiatives in this area. We believe they are urgently needed and will be of great benefit.

Protocols need to be further developed so that active cancer support groups can be repeated like AA groups. The community awareness of this need is just a need to extend cancer support services.

Prevention

It appears that prevention is not a focus of this inquiry. However, the obvious needs to be stated; prevention is better—and easier—than cure.

The Gawler Foundation has a deep commitment to disease prevention, especially cancer prevention. This is achieved largely through promoting a healthy lifestyle based on sound dietary habits, learning life skills such as how to develop and sustain a positive state of mind, stress management, relaxation and meditation.

SUMMARY OF RECOMMENDATIONS

We urge the Committee of inquiry to adopt the following measures:

1. Give acknowledgment to, and affirm the need of patient based, active, cancer support groups.
2. Draw attention to the need for a paradigm shift in the research and treatment of breast cancer. The aim of the successful and

satisfactory management of breast cancer should include the notion that it is gentle on the patient and non invasive. There is a long way to go in this regard. The Inquiry is urged to draw attention to this need.

3. Encourage development of a flexible approach to breast cancer treatment. This approach would ideally include a multi-disciplinary group working as a team with the individual patient's needs as the primary concern.

4. Provide funding support to:
   (i) Individual active cancer support groups.
   (ii) A National Body to coordinate, train and regulate such groups. The Gawler Foundation is helping develop such a body at present; funding is an urgent need to get it established.
   (iii) Individuals—by making support group fees a claimable item on medical benefits.

   The contention is that attending a support group will mean individuals cost the system less and save Government funds.
   (iv) Public Awareness Campaigns. There is an urgent need to raise public awareness to the benefits of self help cancer support groups. A specific campaign would produce great benefit along the lines outlined above in (iii). Secondly, more education is required to convince the public that "Cancer is a word, not a sentence".

5. Instigate change in the relevant State Medical Practitioners Acts to remove the incredible monopoly Doctors hold over the provision of treatment and advice for cancer patients.

6. Instigate specific training for medical students and Post graduate Doctors.
   (i) Communication skills and therapeutic language are urgently needed as a major part of the medical curriculum. Amazingly only a few of Australia's Universities feature such training (Monash and Newcastle being major successful role models). These skills have been

neglected by many of the schools and their deficiency in graduates is often frightening in its negative impact. Such skills are easily taught and urgently required.

(ii) Incorporate closer contact with patients into medical training. Medicine often gives most attention to the "worst" patients—those who are sickest, least responsive, most obscure. More attention should be given to studying "successful" patients—those who recover quickly and/or unexpectedly. This is what we focus on at the Foundation. We can learn a lot from "successful" patients.

(iii) We welcome observers to our programs and regularly have medical staff attend as a learning exercise.

7. Promote Research into Active Cancer Support Groups and Mind/Body Medicine.

(i) A major study is needed to assess the benefits of Australian self help groups. Again as a leader in this field, The Gawler Foundation is keen to cooperate with such research. While we are actively involved in a number of smaller research projects at present, a major study should be instigated and could well focus specifically on women with breast cancer.

(ii) Investigate the cost/benefit ratio of attending an active cancer support group. This would be a great community service.

(iii) Promote the investigation of non toxic gentle therapies. This has been discussed already in the need for a radical shift in the focus of cancer research and treatment.

(iv) Promote open minded research into the benefits, if any, of the real "alternative" treatments. A major problem for many patients is that they hear of improved remedies that have a great appeal and are backed by "anecdotal" evidence. Often patients consider that doctors, particularly oncologists, are unduly biased against these treatments. A more real, major problem is that these treatments will always be there and in the community's best interest, they do need to be fairly evaluated. We propose the establishment of a research body specifically dedicated to uncovering and evaluating innovative, alternative treatments. Presuming this body gained public respect, it could then act as a safeguard as well as a means of introducing worthwhile innovations. Again this is a much needed community service that would have profound benefits.

CONCLUSION

The Gawler Foundation, with its committee of 8, staff of 28, and many voluntary assistants, is dedicated to actively supporting women with breast cancer, as well as other people affected by cancer. We believe that more attention needs to be focused on the patients themselves, rather than the system that exists to treat and support them.

It is evident that more work is required to develop a flexible system that has the resources and staff to meet the individual needs of those women in Australia who are diagnosed with breast cancer and seek help to manage their situation.

We draw particular attention to the need to support cancer support groups because of their unique self help possibilities and the wide ranging benefits they offer to the whole community.

This submission was written by Dr. Ian Gawler, OAM, BVSc. in collaboration with the staff and members of the Gawler Foundation. We would welcome the opportunity to appear before the enquiry if required and would be keen to assist in any way possible to improve the lot of women in Australia, their families and friends, who are affected by breast cancer.

LIST OF APPENDIXES TO THE GAWLER FOUNDATION SUBMISSION

re: Inquiry into the Management and Treatment of Breast Cancer in Australia.

A. Inspiring Personal Profiles—Case histories of people attending The Gawler Foundation's Programs.

B. Cancer patients find strength in self-help approach—Ian Gawler, *Australian Doctor*, 1993.

C. Overview—Breast Cancer, The Gawler Foundation.

D. Patients and their Doctors—What Works, by Ian Gawler. Research presented to the RACGP Conference, Hobart, 1991.

F. Doubts on Breast Treatment, *Australian Doctor* 18/2/94.

F. (i) General Brochure—The Gawler Foundation.
(ii) Details of The Gawler Foundation.

G. The Yarra Valley Cancer Support Group—The Gawler Foundation.

H. The Residential Program—The Gawler Foundation.

I. 142 References for Complementary Medicine and Psychoneuroimmunology—compiled by Ian Gawler, September 1993.

Copies of the above references can be obtained by contacting the Gawler Foundation, P.O. Box 77G, Yarra Junction, 3797, Australia. Telephone (059) 67 1730, Fax (059) 67 1715.

Grace Gawler

Regularly conducts specialized seminars for women dealing with breast cancer. She is General manager and therapist at The Gawler Foundation, Yarra Junction, Victoria, Australia.

Grace, and her husband Ian, facilitate this unique international centre which is a non-profit, non-denominational, charitable organisation.

The Foundation is well recognised for its support and education programs in the area of cancer management. Recognising the need for prevention of illness and the promotion of wellbeing. The Foundation also conducts meditation, stress management, and healthy lifestyle seminars. Personal counselling is available.

Regular seminars and residential programs are conducted in all areas of health care. The Foundation houses a specialist book and tape shop, catering for all the needs of patients and their families in dealing with cancer.

Write or ring for a book and tape brochure or general service information.

Help is just a phone call away!

If you feel we can help you—reach out and ring or write to:

The Gawler Foundation
P.O. Box 77G
Yarra Junction
Victoria, 3797, Australia

General Enquiries:	**Phone:**	**(059) 67 1730**
Seminar Information:	**Phone:**	**(059) 67 2232**
	Fax:	**(059) 67 1715**